BIG THIGHS

CHOCOLATE CUPCAKES

AND MY FIRST KISS

Poppie Pie and The Yum Yum Club

Suzanne Brown, RD

This book is dedicated my nutty family!

With heaping thanks to my teenage daughter who did unsuccessfully microwave oatmeal at age four and has successfully created lovely meals since, and to my teenage son who amused himself as a toddler smelling all the cooking spices and later taught himself to make migas, and to my hubbie who has put his heart and love into cooking incredible meals for me since our second date so many years ago.

I love that we all cook together. I love every morsel, every snort of laughter and every floury handprint, and that all of you are willing to try my recipe tweaks.
Thank you!

CONTENTS

CHAPTER 1

A Bully in Papa's Café

My name is Poppie, and I'm huge.

There. I said it.

I'm a huge, towering giant who loves potato chips, cookies, gummy worms, and orange soda. I grew up on mac and cheese, frozen pizza, and anything else that could be warmed up in a microwave or carried out in a to-go bag.

I eat like crap, but I can also snowboard black moguls, ace geometry, and slam dunk a basketball better than most boys in my high school.

But none of that matters a flip when you're fat. Because boys don't kiss fat girls. Especially this one.

I would love my first kiss to happen before my skin wrinkles up like a walnut so my best friend, Kale, and I are on our way to a healthy cooking class. On the first day of Christmas break. When we should be shredding fresh powder and making our lists for Santa.

Why am I doing this again?

I stop on the sidewalk and try to convince myself that this is a great idea. "I'm almost eighty-seven percent certain I will get my first kiss if I lose twenty pounds."

Kale doesn't stop walking. He's heard this before. He doesn't agree.

"Dude!" I jog to catch up. "I mean it. I think twenty pounds is my magic number. Like princess-in-a-fairy-tale magic where the prince is a total hottie."

Kale shakes his head. "Pass."

I laugh. "Fine. How long until class starts?"

"Why?"

I gesture to the slope, all sparkly with fresh snow. "Just wondering if we have time for a quick ride."

We live in Butte, Colorado. Elevation: 8,700 feet. We have one main street, one grocery store, and one world-class ski resort called The Rock. It's smaller than Vail or Breckenridge, but has three chair lifts, 25 runs, and I think some of the best snow in the Rocky Mountains. Especially today.

Kale gazes up at The Rock and his brown eyes glaze over. "That was a radical dump last night," he mumbles. "Probably 8 inches."

I nod in encouragement. "Yeah."

"And it is a sick day."

"The best." I grin. I like where this is going.

Kale and I met at ski school when we were six. I pushed him down the bunny hill and told him he could fly. He couldn't, so I felt really bad and shared my brownie with him. Since his parents are health nuts and never let him eat sugar, he quickly forgave me and we've been besties ever since. We look as different as salt and pepper with his dark licorice skin and charcoal rotini hair and my floury white skin and stringy-as-coconut hair, but I bring out the silly in him and he puts up with me, so we're a great match.

Kale is still weighing options. "The forecast is projecting increasing temps which means the snow could be too slushy this afternoon, making the conditions ideal at the present moment. If we take Bluebird to Dark Horse, we can be up in 7 minutes and down in…" He sighs and shakes his head. "We just don't have enough time. Class starts in fifteen minutes."

I roll my eyes. Kale is a rule-following overachiever. I don't know why I hang out with him.

"We could be late," I whisper.

Kale arches an eyebrow. "You hate being late."

He's right, but I roll my eyes again anyway.

He grins. "The Rock will still be here when class is over."

"Yeah," I grumble, "three days from now."

He raises both ebony eyebrows. "I distinctly remember some girl that sounds just like you begging me to take this cooking class with her. And now you don't want to go?"

Oh yeah. That's why I hang out with him. Because he puts up with me.

I look at The Rock and then back at Kale. I want a boy to kiss me. So, I need to lose twenty pounds. Which means I need to learn to cook something besides mac and cheese. I need this cooking class.

I blow the mountain a kiss. "Sorry to break your heart, big guy, but we can't hang out right now." I nudge Kale. "Thanks for coming with me."

He shrugs, the neon green spikes on his ski hat bobbing back and forth. "You know I'm just in it for the cookies."

I laugh. "I know. Me, too."

We walk another half block until we reach Papa's Market where the class is being held. The building is gray weathered wood with a colorful rainbow arching over the revolving front door. Papa Shortdough opened his market way before I was born, and it's a staple in our little town. Papa's Market is a favorite for locals and a must-see for tourists. He always has something for everyone. Fresh produce all year long. Hard to find spices and herbs. Camping foods. Hot cocoa and coffee in the winter, iced in the summer. Warm, homemade bread. Fresh sandwiches. And his famous cookies.

Kale heads into the market. For some reason, I don't follow. I think my snow boots must have frozen to the ground. Or maybe I'm afraid that after this class I might never see a taco again.

When Kale notices I'm not behind him, he turns to the window and yells, "Purr going boo kiss tall the wookies!"

I make a face at him. "What?"

He cups his hands around his mouth and yells louder. "You're going to miss all the cookies!"

I press my lips on the window like a fat fish. He smacks the window and I jump back laughing.

He grins. "Guess that means more cookies for me!"

I know he means it, so I jump into the revolving door, but instead of popping out into the market, I wave to Kale and continue revolving past him. A rush of cool air blasts me when the door passes the street. A small part of me wants to flee, but I stay and push harder. I see Kale grin as I pass him in the market. I keep revolving and soon I'm spinning so fast that I have to run to keep up. The sidewalk speeds by in a blur. Kale is a blur. I smell crisp snow. Then warm chocolate and fresh bread. Snow. Chocolate. Bread. Snow! Chocolate! Bread! I'm spinning so fast that I feel like my freckles are going to fly off my face and I'm so dizzy with happy that I never want to stop.

Then Kale starts waving his arms at me. He looks a bit panicked, so I slow a bit to see why. He points to a guy waiting outside on the snowy sidewalk.

I shake my head. "Can't stop!" I yell as I pass him. Wonder how many times I would have to revolve to set a world record?

WHAM! The door suddenly slams to a stop. My hands prevent my body from crashing into the glass, but I'm jarred out of my euphoria. NO! My world record! Gone.

I square my shoulders and inhale a deep breath. That's okay. New plan. I'll just start again. I push the door. It doesn't budge. I shove my body weight against it. Nothing. I twist my head around and spot the problem. The guy outside has shoved his snowboard boot into the door.

I frown. "Move your boot!" I yell.

"You groove!" he yells back.

I tilt my head. "You want me to dance?"

He shakes his head, cups his hands around his mouth, and

yells, "Move!"

I giggle. Oh. That makes more sense.

WHAM! The door suddenly starts moving, propelling me forward. The heel of my boot gets stuck which throws me off balance and spits me out into the market, careening straight towards Kale.

"Aeeeeii!" I exclaim, arms flapping, stumbling like the floor is covered in banana peels. I smash into Kale, bounce off his chest, and we both tumble to the floor.

A few people look concerned, but the regulars don't even look up. They know Kale and me.

"Dude, that was sweet!" I squeal.

Kale is lying next to me, flat on his back, looking like roadkill. "Oh yeah," he groans. "Sweet."

I notice the guy from outside is walking towards us holding my boot. He looks a little older than us, and for some odd reason, he's dressed all in black. Black ski hat. Black coat. Black jeans. Black, world-record-crushing, snowboarding boots. Which oddly he's wearing in a store! He stops right next to my head. I expect him to apologize, or offer me a hand up, or at the very least give our acrobatics a perfect ten, but instead he just gawks at my boot like it's a mutant.

"I'm assuming this is yours?" he asks, dropping the boot so close to my face that I flinch. "Your feet must be huge!"

No. He did not.

I ball my hands into fists. No. One. Calls. Me. Huge.

He tilts his head. "I think we may wear the same huge size."

That's it. I know a bully when I see one.

I start to laugh, quietly at first, and then louder until I'm basically shrieking. A few customers throw their hands over their ears so I figure I must be hitting some really good notes.

"Oh, dude," I chuckle. "You are *so* funny."

My mom once told me laughter is a good way to deal with bullies because they never know what to do when their mean remarks don't hurt. Something about taking the steam out of the bull.

I nudge Kale who's still lying next to me like a dead fish. "Isn't he just *so* funny?"

Kale raises an eyebrow at me, and shakes his head. He's not playing.

"Whatevs," our new friend mumbles and removes his sunglasses.

I try not to laugh. His face is beyond sunburned except for the glaring white circles around his eyes. Normally I wouldn't stoop so low as to make fun of someone's appearance, but I like to make an exception for jerks who ruin my world record attempt, almost drop a boot on my face, and call me huge.

I give him my best pity smile. "Looks like you got a nasty burn from that big ball of fire in the sky we like to call the sun." I giggle. "Welcome to Colorado, Red."

"Whatevs," he mutters, shakes his head, and walks away.

I stand up and give him a little finger wave. "See you around, Red."

Oddly, he doesn't wave back.

Kale stands up and brushes off his pants. "Red?"

"Thought it was a cute nickname for such a friendly fellow," I giggle, "who looks like Santa's very helpful red-nosed reindeer."

Kale laughs. "You're a goof."

I grab my boot and shove my foot into it. "Always."

Kale checks his watch. "Although that was riveting fun, I want a cookie before class starts."

I nod, and lead us past the front of Papa's Market where there's a small grocery and a long, wooden counter facing out the window where people can sit and eat their sandwiches or sip their cocoa while looking at The Rock Ski Resort across the street. Then we pass a cozy area stuffed with deep couches and red velvet armchairs near the huge fireplace. Everyone loves lingering in these two areas of Papa's Market.

But not Kale and me.

We love the back of the market where there's a small

horseshoe-shaped counter facing the open kitchen. The counter is covered in black-and-white checkerboard tile and surrounded by six, metal stools with shiny, red, plastic seats. Kale and I love hanging out back here after school. Mainly because of the cookies. But also because we get to see Papa. And Papa is pretty cool.

I throw my backpack on the floor and bounce onto a barstool. My jeans charm a loud squeal from the plastic seat.

Kale slides onto the stool next to me without making a sound. He jumps off, purses his lips, and slides on again. This time he gets a loud *FWAAAP*. I put my hand over my mouth and act shocked. Kale fist pumps the air. This is why we're best friends.

I shrug out of my orange fleece and stuff it under my stool, while Kale carefully lays his green jacket over the back of his stool.

He turns back to me and sticks out his chest, showing off his tie. "What do you think?"

A few months ago when we started as lowly freshman in high school, Kale thought he could loosen up his image by wearing one of his dad's old ties every day. No one really wears ties anymore, so I'm not sure it's changing his image but he likes it so I do, too. Today he's wearing a red tie covered with vibrant purple Christmas trees.

I give it a thumbs up. "Very cool." I point to the purple cartoon reindeer on my shirt. "And it matches Rudolphia Lightenhousen." Which I think is a perfect name for a reindeer with a bulbous red nose, a huge toothy grin, and a speech bubble that reads:

I know I'm different, but I let my light shine anyway.

We're interrupted by a loud voice snapping, "This will be my last offer."

I widen my eyes. "I wonder who's back there with Papa," I whisper.

Kale shrugs and opens his mouth to reply but immediately closes it when he sees Papa Shortdough walk out of his kitchen followed by a man wearing a dark business suit.

"I mean it," The Suit warns in a voice so arrogant and menacing that I get goosebumps. He's tall and lean, and obviously well-dressed, but his dark hair is plastered across his forehead in an odd angle covering one of his beady, little eyes.

"Awesome," Papa Shortdough replies with a nod. "Then I won't have to tell you no again."

"You will be sorry you ripped up his offer," the suit scolds, and when Papa doesn't reply, he smooths an errant piece of hair from his cheek, and calmly walks away.

Papa watches him stalk through the market and out the door before letting out a big sigh. We're sitting on the opposite side of the room so I don't think Papa knows we're here so I Clear my throat to get his attention.

He glances over, surprised to see us. "Hey," he bellows. "How are my favorite shredders?"

Papa Shortdough is an aging mix of mountain man, health food nut, and bodybuilder. He's short, completely bald, and always wears starched, button-down shirts, jeans, and an apron. He's bursting with ripped muscles and skis better than me or any of my friends, but is old enough to be my grandpa. He looks like a wrinkled bulldog that could rip out your throat, but he's actually the sweetest dude in the whole world, and I adore him.

I notice his killer smile doesn't quite reach his crinkly eyes today. I wonder if that has something to do with The Suit.

I nod my head towards the door. "What's up with the stiff?" I know no boundaries.

Papa shrugs. "Eh. He's just doing his job. I wouldn't worry about him."

But Papa looks worried, and that bothers me.

He lowers his elbows onto the counter and grins. "Ready?"

Kale and I get into position. Elbows secure on the counter. Fists up.

"Set?" Papa thunders. His muscular arms bulge above his splattered apron as he raises his cannonball fists and latches onto our hands.

"And go!" Papa bellows, marking the beginning of a thumb war. It's our thing with Papa. We do it every day when we get to the market. Our version of a hug, I guess.

I fling my thumb around as fast as I can, but Papa quickly crushes it under his meaty one. I glance over and see he's flattened Kale's, too.

I pretend to pout. "You always win."

Papa chuckles and tugs one of my long braids. "Only because I have years of practice."

"Nice moves, Mr. Shortdough."

Ugh. It's our bully buddy, Red. And he's walking out of the kitchen. What was *he* doing back there?

I see he's traded his snowboarding boots for black cowboy boots, but his face is still sunburned, and unless he's had a life-changing experience in the past five minutes, I imagine he's still a jerk.

Red arches an eyebrow. "Want some stiffer competition than these kids?"

Kids? I bite my tongue, and try really hard not to roll my eyes. What is it with him?

Papa has barely latched onto Red's fingers when Red tries to catch him off guard and shouts, "Ready, set, go!"

I almost laugh at Red's feeble attempt at cheating because before he can even move his thumb Papa has captured it. I cheer, Kale whoops, and Red just looks... well, more red.

Papa slaps Red on the back. "Don't sweat it. Maybe next time." He wiggles his thumb in our direction. "Nick, meet Poppie and Kale."

As Nick spreads his chapped lips into a forced grin, I hold out my hand.

"Charmed."

Red grits his teeth, but shakes my hand. "Nice to meet you," he says politely, and then frowns when Papa ducks his head under the counter.

I very maturely stick out my tongue.

He squeezes my hand.

I squeeze his even harder.

Papa straightens back up and sets napkins on the counter. "Nick is helping me with the cooking class."

I drop Nick's hand, and have a heart attack. "Red's doing what?" I blurt before I can stop myself.

Kale kicks me. Nick glares at me. And Papa gives me a funny look.

"Who's Red?"

Oops. Would you believe it was Rudolph?

CHAPTER 2

It's December, Not February!

"**R**ed?" I shake my head and laugh. "Did I say Red?"

Papa raises one bushy, white eyebrow, and nods.

I giggle. "Oh, silly, silly me. I meant to say Nick, but I was thinking of Ned from this book I was reading so I must have mixed the two up. Nick. Ned. Red. All so similar!" I twirl one of my braids proving my innocence. "Although I really like Red. Maybe people should start calling you that? I could start a new trend?" I really like being helpful.

Nick is gritting his teeth so hard that I'm afraid his head might pop off.

"No," he grumbles. "Nick is just fine."

Papa glances at Nick, and then at me, and then back at Nick. He narrows his eyes. "Is something going on here that I should know about?"

Nick shakes his head. "No, sir."

Papa looks at me.

I grin. "All good here." I rest my elbows on the counter and place my chin in my hands. "How are things with you, Papa?"

Papa adds more wrinkles to his forehead and looks like he's about to lecture us, but instead he just shakes his head.

"Okay. I don't believe either of you for a minute, but I'll let it go." He motions to Nick. "Come on back into the kitchen, I need to show you something before class starts."

I wait until they disappear before I grab Kale's arm. "Mister ruin-my-world-record and wants-to-kill-me-with-my-boot is helping with the cooking class?!" I shriek.

Kale raises one dark eyebrow. "Kill you with your boot?"

"This is a disaster!" I throw my arm across my forehead like I've seen those frail ladies do in my grandma's movies when they're faced with a tragedy. I wonder if I'm supposed to faint now.

I sigh. "There's no way I'm going to learn anything from him. He's a bully, and he's mean, and he didn't say he was sorry for shattering my word record attempt, and … and…" I plunk my forehead onto the counter. "He's not Papa Shortdough."

Kale pats my back like I'm a child throwing a tantrum, which I kind of am.

"Maybe it won't be so bad," he says. "Papa said Nick was *helping*. That means Papa is still teaching us."

I know Kale is right, but it doesn't make me any happier. I'd love to leave and forget the whole thing. I mean, who really cares if I lose weight? Fat is in. Huge is cool. Big is boss.

I groan. Who am I kidding? No boy wants to kiss a girl who's six feet tall, and chunky as peanut butter and jiggly as gravy.

My dad played hockey at university and my mom's ancestors were Vikings, so big is definitely in my genes. But I'm a smart girl. I know why I have a little chubb in the tub. I eat like crap. Cheesy puffs. Gummy worms. French fries. Tacos. Donuts. Pepperoni pizza. Add an orange soda, and dinner is served!

Yep. I'm a jumbo-sized, junk food addict.

I may love junk food more than my snowboard. Maybe even more than my cell phone. And definitely more than my science teacher, Mrs. Finklepop, who freaked me out last week when she went on and on about heart disease.

Yeah. Heart disease. I'm barely a freshman in high school

and now I'm worried about having a heart attack!

Muchos gracias, Mrs. F.

Since I eat tons of junk food and my family eats takeout every night, I got a little worried about all of us keeling over, so I cooked dinner that night. I made spaghetti thinking it would be so easy. Cook noodles. Open jar of sauce. Voila! Dinner is served.

It wasn't that easy. I burned it.

I made scrambled eggs and toast the next night.

Burned them.

Frozen pizza. Burned. Chicken nuggets. Blackened.

You see where I'm going here.

My family wouldn't stop teasing me about burning everything to a crisp, so I blew up and promised to prove that I can cook by making the best Christmas Eve dinner they've ever had that they would be so sorry for teasing me.

And now I'm sorry. Because I never go back on a promise, and although I have no idea how to cook an entire Christmas Eve dinner, I will not admit defeat. I need to prove to myself, and my family, that I can do it. I can make Christmas Eve dinner. I can lose twenty pounds. I can find a boy to kiss me.

So, I guess I need this class.

Unless I'm lucky enough to catch the chicken pox in the next few minutes, or a bunch of people wearing wetsuits walk in and desperately need me to leave now for Antarctica to help them study penguins.

Papa taps my shoulder with his beefy fingers. "Poppie, what are you doing?"

I lift my head up and manage a smile. "Chin push-ups?"

He sets a towel-covered tray down on the counter, and frowns at me. "Poppie."

I sigh. "Well, the thing is that I just remembered that I burn everything I cook, so instead of totally ruining your class, I think you should nicely kick me out and send me home."

Papa chuckles. "Now why would I do that? Poppie anyone can be a chef. Even you."

I snort. "Yeah. Chef Burn."

He laughs. "I don't know about that, but I do know that if you leave now, you won't get to have one of these." He reaches down and flicks the towel off the tray, revealing colossal chocolate cookies, bursting with white and dark chocolate chips.

"You made Triple-Chocolate Cookies!" I shout.

My woes disappear in a poof and the world instantly becomes a happy place again. *Papa's Triple-Chocolate Cookies* have that power. No joke.

Papa is the only one who knows how to make these cookies. He guards the secret recipe handed down from his great-great-great-great-great grandmother like the world's existence depends on it. Which it probably does. Because once you taste one of *Papa's Triple-Chocolate Cookies* it would be the end of the world to never get another.

Papa points to two cookies that are much bigger than the others. "I'd pick those if I were you," he says with a wink before bustling back into the kitchen.

My mouth starts watering. I grab one of the big ones, inhale the glorious scent of warm chocolate, and take a huge bite. A chocolate fudge cookie, crisp on the edges and gooey soft in the middle. How does he do that? It's perfect. The melty white and dark chocolate chips coat my mouth and make me feel like I'm snuggling under a soft blanket on a snowy, winter night.

I'm just about to chomp another sigh-inducing bite when the sugar hits my brain. "Wait a minute. It's not February."

Kale raises one eyebrow as he swallows. "Um, no."

"It's December twenty-second, right?"

"Yeah."

I grab Kale's arm. "We're eating *Papa's Triple-Chocolate Cookies*, and it's not February!" I narrow my eyes and glare into the kitchen. "Something's not right. Papa only makes these cookies on my birthday."

Kale corrects me with a grin. "I'm pretty sure he makes them for Valentine's Day."

I wave him off. "My birthday. Valentines. Whatever. It's the same day. But it's the only day Papa ever makes these cookies."

I always have *Papa's Triple-Chocolate Cookies* on my birthday with a big candle stuck in the center. A blizzard almost broke my streak last February when it rudely dumped five-feet of snow in one day. Five feet! Even a ski resort can't handle that much snow that fast. The plows couldn't keep the roads Clear, and everyone was stuck in their houses. I thought for sure it would be my first birthday ever without *Papa's Triple-Chocolate Cookies*, and I was devastated. But then guess who showed up at my front door, wearing snowshoes, a crinkly grin, and a backpack of warm cookies. Yep. Papa.

I really do adore him.

"It doesn't make sense," I explain to Kale. "Papa can only get that special chocolate from Transylvania in February."

Kale snickers. "Transylvania? Do vampires make it?" He licks his fingers. "I think you mean Slovenia."

I pound my fist on the counter. "EXACTLY! So how did he make them today?"

Kale shrugs. "Leftover chocolate?"

I make a buzzing sound. "Bzzz! Wrong! Sorry, that answer is incorrect. Papa told me the chocolate only stays fresh for a week."

Papa walks out of the kitchen and sets two glasses of milk on the counter. The glasses are frosted and icy cold just like always.

"Thanks, Papa," I say and take a quick gulp. I set my glass down and rub my hands together. "Now it's time for you to give us some answers."

Papa raises his bushy white eyebrows. "Answers?"

I place my palms on the counter. "It's not Valentine's Day."

"Or Poppie's birfday," Kale adds through a mouthful of cookie.

I lean over the counter until I'm nose-to-nose with Papa Shortdough. I scrunch my face into what I think is a bad-cop grimace. "So, just *how* were you able to make these cookies today?"

Papa Shortdough winks. "Can't tell you."

"Tough nut to crack, eh?" I decide to try good-cop. I sit back down on my stool, twirl one of my braids, and smile. "We sure would love to know. Pretty please!"

Papa shakes his head. "Nope."

Kale tries to help me. "Did you make them for something special?"

That makes Papa grins wider than I do on Christmas morning when I see all my presents under the tree. "Enjoy the cookies," he sings and does a weird step-dance back into the kitchen.

I narrow my eyes. "Something is definitely up."

Kale shrugs. "I guess so."

"Why won't he tell us why he made them today?"

Kale gulps the last of his milk and wipes his mouth. "Guess it's a secret."

I pause with the last bite of cookie melting in my hand.

A secret? Papa Shortdough has a secret?

Well, deck the halls with boughs of holly.

CHAPTER 3

Secrets and Soccer and Smile Hour

P apa Shortdough has a secret.

Sweet! I love secrets! Mainly because I love unearthing the nitty gritty details.

I'm busy concocting a Poppie-licious plan when a boy I vaguely recognize walks up to the counter. He's wearing a ski hat with some sort of crest on it and the letters FCB.

"Is this where meet *Yum Yum*?" he asks in a thick accent.

Kale extends his hand. "Yea. I'm Kale and this is Poppie. We're taking the class, too."

I wave. "Hey, dude. I'm Poppie Pie Sunshine Wellington."

His eyes widen.

Kale rolls his eyes. "You can just call her Poppie."

The boy's mouth curls into a grin. "I think this will be fun class." He sits on the stool next to Kale, removes his ski hat, and runs his hand through his wavy, brown hair. Wow. No hat head for his gorgeous, thick waves. Me and my straight-up frizz are jealous.

He extends his hand. "I am Ignacio Martín Alvarez Vilanova Casillas." I think he sees my mouth drop open because he winks and adds, "But friends call me Nacho."

"Do you go to BHS?" Kale asks.

Nacho's mouth twists in confusion. "BHS?"

I explain. "Butte High School." Then I suddenly remember why he looks familiar. "You were playing soccer at lunch yesterday!"

Nacho pauses a second, scrunches his eyebrows together and then smiles. "Yes, soccer. I was playing soccer." He puts his hands out in front of him, palms up. "Sorry, where I'm from we call fútbol."

"Where are you from?" Kale asks.

"Barcelona. In España." Nacho shakes his head. His cocoa waves don't move. "Um, sorry. You call Spain. I am exchange student. I arrive week ago. And now I take this class so I can eat."

A girl bundled up in a thick scarf, ski mask, and what looks like a coat way too big for her body stops at the stool next to Nacho. As soon as she takes off her ski mask, I recognize her from my AP World Geography class at school.

I lean forward and wave in her direction. "Hey, Clea!"

She mumbles a soft "Hello" through a veil of long, black hair, never looking up as she unwinds her scarf and sets it on the stool. She unzips her gray coat, shrugs out of it, and sets it on top of the scarf. Then she unzips another coat, takes it off, and adds it to her pile of clothes. Clea rarely talks, but I do know she's super shy and moved this summer from a little Caribbean island called Dominica. With all the layers she's wearing, I'm thinking she may still be adjusting to the cold.

"Hey, Clea," Kale says. "Are you here for *Yum Yum*?"

Clea nods. She's big like me, but way shorter. My guess is she wants to lose weight, too.

Kale motions to Nacho. "This is Nacho. He's taking the class, too." Before Clea has time to nod again, Kale turns back to Nacho and shakes his head. "Wait a minute! You said you have to take this class so you can eat? Isn't your host family supposed to feed you?"

Nacho looks concerned. "Maybe I not say that right?" He taps his chin. "My English is sometimes not good. I take this class to eat because my host family not eat real food."

I laugh. "They don't eat real food? Are they zombies?" I lean forward. "Do you still have all your fingers? I hear they nibble on those first."

Nacho laughs. "My host family have not eat my fingers." He shows me all ten of his fingers. "They are allergic to much foods, and the foods they eat," he makes a face, "they not taste very good. I don't complain because they are so nice." He pauses to rub his belly. "But I'm starving!"

"Hallo!" a shrill voice calls out from behind us.

Without even turning around, I know it's Tiffany Bouffe, the most popular girl at our school. Or at least she thinks she is. No one really likes her snotty personality, but everyone wants to be her friend because her parents own C'est La Ski, the only restaurant at the bottom of the ski slope.

Tiffany bounces her petite, perfectly-sized body over to Nacho, and I wonder why in the world she's here. She places her hand on Nacho's arm. "If you're starving, handsome, you should come eat at my restaurant." She flutters her big brown eyes, tosses back her glossy brown hair in that way popular girls seem born to do, and then smiles her megawatt grin.

"Um, thank you," Nacho says politely.

Tiffany waves her hand in the air. "Anytime." She looks over at Clea, then back at Nacho, and then back at Clea. I can't see Tiffany's face, but I'm betting she has narrowed her eyes and pursed her lips. I've seen her do it before in the cafeteria when someone is sitting at her table.

Clea drops her head, stands up, and starts collecting all her clothing off the stool. Without a word of thanks, Tiffany sits down on what used to be Clea's stool, and faces Nacho. She's wearing a pink sweater that looks like a lot of cotton candy gave their lives to make.

"Now, I believe you were just about to ask me to dinner, Nacho?"

Instead of sitting back down, Clea starts walking toward the front door. Nope. This is not happening. I jump up and catch up to her.

"Where ya going?" I ask.

She glances back at Tiffany, and then stares at the ground. "I just don't think this is a good idea."

I flip my hand in Tiffany's direction. "Aw, who cares about her? If you..."

I pause. Wait a minute! This is my golden opportunity. A good friend would never let Clea leave all by herself. A good friend would go with her to keep her company.

And I am a good friend.

I link my arm through Clea's and pull her toward the door. "What I meant was if you leave, I'll go with you!"

We've almost reached the revolving door of freedom (and no Nick!) when Li Xiu Ying walks into the café. At six-one, Li is a little taller than me, co-captain of the girls' varsity soccer team (as a freshman!), and friends with everyone. Her brown, almond-shaped eyes are always lined with silver, her black hair is always cropped in a short pixie, and her ears are always sporting dangling earrings.

"Yo!" Li greets us with a smile as silver snowmen bob from her ears. "Are you doing the yumster class, too?"

I want to say no and pull Clea out the door, but I can't lie, especially to the nicest girl in the world.

I nod. "Yep."

"Cool!" Li links one arm through mine, the other through Clea's, and drags us both back to the counter.

I slide back onto my stool. Li sits next to me and Clea sits next to her.

Li leans around me. "Yo, Kale! Tiffany!" She grins wide at Nacho. "Nacho man, that was some move yesterday during the fútbol game."

Nacho grins back. "Not cool as your header!"

"At least it's good for something!" Li laughs and knocks on her head.

This makes everyone laugh because we all know Li is one of the smartest kids in our class. Tiffany is the only one not laughing. I don't think she likes that Nacho is paying attention to someone besides her.

Tiffany puts her hand on Nacho's arm. "You must tell me your favorite place to shop in Barcetown?"

Nacho shakes his head. "Sorry. Where is this Barcetown?"

Tiffany yaps her yippy dog laugh. "Hee hee hee!" She playfully slaps his arm. "You're so silly. Barcetown. Like, where you live in Spain!"

Li laughs. "Yo, girlfriend, you mean Barcelona." And Li actually pronounces it Bar-*thee*-lona, just like Nacho does.

Tiffany furrows her brow. "You live in Barcelona?"

Nacho nods. "Yes. And I'm sorry but I not shop much." He turns back to Li. "You watch Messi last night?"

"You bet I did!" Li punches the air. "What a move!" She shakes her head. "Sorry, everyone. Messi plays fútbol for FC Barcelona." She leans back to try to include Clea in the conversation and points to the blue and red striped shirt that Nacho is wearing. It has the same initials - FCB - as his hat. "They're Nacho's home team and last night Messi..."

"I know. I know," Tiffany interrupts in a huff, obviously upset that she's not the center of attention. "He's going to the Super Bowl."

Everyone bursts out laughing. Even Clea cracks a smile.

Tiffany puckers her lips. "What?"

Nacho tries to look serious. "This is not the American football. fútbol teams do not go to the Super Bowl."

Nacho starts explaining about soccer teams competing in the World Cup, but I stop listening when a blur in the kitchen catches my eye, and I realize the blur is Nick. He dashes across the kitchen and hides behind a tall rack. What in the world? I lean back to get a better view. Is he spying on us? I wonder if anyone else sees him, but Li is talking to Clea, Kale and Nacho have their heads back howling in laughter, and Tiffany is yawning. I turn back just in time to see Nick skirt around the far edge of the counter and sprint towards the door.

Kale waves his hand in front of my face. "Earth to Poppie. Isn't that right?"

I shake my head. Ok, that was weird.

"Sorry, zoned out for a sec," I apologize. "What's right?"

"In Barcelona, we eat dinner very late, at eleven," Nacho explains. "So, we eat tapas around five. Americans say appetizers, but Kale says you call *Smile Hour Appie*."

I grin. "He's right. I do. Because eating food always makes me smile."

"Well said, Poppie," Papa booms as he emerges from the kitchen. He grins. "And nothing makes me smile more than seeing all of you here." He extends out his bulging arms. "Welcome everyone to our first *Yum Yum* class." He nods hello to everyone. "Tiffany. Nacho. Kale. Poppie. Li." When he reaches Clea he bows slightly. "And I'm sorry but I haven't had the pleasure of making your acquaintance, young lady." He extends his hand. "I'm Papa Shortdough."

Clea reaches out her hand, but doesn't look up. "I'm Clea," she says softly.

Instead of shaking her hand and letting go, he latches onto it. She looks up startled and tries to pull her hand away, but Papa merely raises one bushy white eyebrow.

"You ready?"

"Ready?" Clea asks.

I laugh. "When you shake hands with Papa, you have a thumb war."

A hint of a smile forms on Clea's lips. "A thumb war?"

Papa nods with a grin. "You ready?"

"Um, ok," Clea says slowly.

"Set," Papa says.

They both raise their thumbs.

"And go!"

I'm shocked when Papa doesn't immediately win. The two of them battle on, thumbs wriggling frantically. Clea bites her lip. Sweat beads on Papa's bicep. Then to everyone's utter surprise Clea shoves Papa Shortdough's thumb under hers.

Li jumps up and raises Clea's arm in the air. "The winnah!"

Everyone claps and shouts congratulations, while Tiffany

just sits there staring at her nails.

I lean around Li and slap Clea on the back. "Way to go! No one ever beats Papa! How'd you do that?"

Clea tucks one side of her hair behind her ear. "Lots of practice with my four brothers." She shrugs. "It's the only way our parents let us fight."

Papa laughs. "Smart parents. And you're definitely the best opponent I've ever had." He winks. "Great job, young lady. You'll have to teach me your strategy someday."

Clea immediately blushes and pulls her hair back in front of her face.

Papa claps his hands. "Okay, then. I have three days to transform you all into chefs, so let's get started." He makes a fist and presses it over his heart. "I promise that no matter your skill level, you will all learn to cook healthy and fabulously tasty food by the end of this class." He motions behind us. "And this is my assistant, Nick. He'll be here to help you learn, too."

Everyone turns around. Nick holds up two fingers in a peace sign, looking way more relaxed than he did when he was hiding behind shelves a few minutes before.

"What's up?" Nick says coolly.

Tiffany is the only one who seems impressed. "Oh, hallo, Nick," she coos, fluttering her eyelashes. "What's *your* favorite thing to cook?"

Nick leans closer to her, and grins. "Anything sweet."

I groan. This is going to be a long three days. Maybe I should go take a walk in the winter wonderland.

CHAPTER 4

Watch Out for Undies in the Fridge

P apa Shortdough leans against the counter. "Before we get started, who has cooked before?"

We all raise our hands.

Papa smiles. "Great! Then we can skip some basics and dive right in. Class starts every day at ten and should finish by two. Today we'll make breakfast, tomorrow lunch, and then our grand finale on Christmas Eve will be dinner." He throws a quick wink my way. He knows that's why I'm here. I didn't tell him about the kiss and the twenty pounds.

Papa pulls out a pile of aprons and sets them on the counter. "Everyone please put on an apron. Ladies," he pauses, glances at Kale's shoulder-length curls and adds, "and Kale, please make certain your hair is back in a ponytail or in braids like Poppie's."

Kale plops his green ski hat back on his head. He grabs the neon green spikes on top and wraps them in a ponytail. He smiles. "This good?"

Papa chortles. "Yes. That'll work."

Li raises her hand. "Am I okay Papa Shortdough?" she asks, pointing to her short hair.

He nods. "Yep. You're fine." He looks at Clea. "Guess it's

just you, Champ. Hair back, please."

Everyone stands up and heads around the counter to grab an apron. I notice Clea is still sitting on her stool searching through her coats.

"Everything ok?" I ask.

She looks up at me with that one eye peeking through her hair. "I don't think I have a ponytail holder," she whispers, sounding like she's about to cry.

I take the extra one I always keep on my wrist and hand it to her. "I do. Here."

"You sure you don't need it?"

"Nah. I always carry an extra."

She exhales with relief. "Thanks."

She pulls her hair over to the side of her head and ties it up into a bun. I'm pretty sure this is the first time I've seen her face not covered by her hair. Her brown eyes are almost the same color as her caramel skin.

I give her a thumbs up. "Cool bun."

Her face flushes pink, but I see a tiny smile curl her lips. "Thanks."

We skirt around the counter, grab our aprons, and hurry through the kitchen to catch up to the rest of the group. We find them in the back standing around a silver counter.

Papa hands out packets of paper. "Here are the recipes for today. This will be our prep area, but first we need to collect our ingredients. Everyone follow me." He leads us deeper into the kitchen, and stops in front of a large, silver door that's twice as tall and twice as wide as him.

"This is the walk-in fridge. Poppie, Clea, and Nacho, please gather the cold ingredients and bring them to the workstation. Kale, Li, and Tiffany, follow me. I'll show you where to collect the dry ingredients."

As they walk away, I turn to Clea and Nacho and punch my fist in the air. "Go, Team Refrigerator!" I throw my arms around their shoulders and pull them into a huddle. "Here's the plan. If we zigzag back and throw the pass, the door may never see us coming and we can get inside!"

They both stare at me for a heartbeat and I wonder if I need to dial back the crazy, but then Clea claps her hands together and says, "Break!"

Well, look at that! Clea has a sense of humor behind all that hair. Who would have known?

She points over my head. "Go long!"

I turn around, run a few feet, and swivel back towards her just as she tosses her packet of recipes to me.

"Quick!" I yell to Nacho. "While it's distracted! Open the door!"

Nacho grins, dashes over to the door, grabs the shiny metal handle and pulls it open.

WHOOSH!

I high-five Clea, and return her packet.. I strut over to where Nacho is holding the door open. "Good work, Ignacio Martín Alvarez Vilanova Casillas."

He looks surprised that I remembered his entire name, but then answers, "Thank you, Poppie Pie Sunshine Wellington."

"Nice!" I laugh. Maybe this class won't be so bad after all.

I step into the fridge and a rush of cold air envelops me. It isn't very deep, but it's big enough that when Clea and Nacho follow me in, there's still plenty of room for us to move around.

I glance at the ingredients listed on the packet. "First, a dozen eggs."

Nacho grabs an egg carton from the shelf. "Got it."

I look down for the next ingredient just as the door closes, the lights go out, and we're plunged into blackness.

Great. I hate it when I get shut into a refrigerator and the lights go out because that's when the giant underwear appears.

Let me explain.

I once had this truly bizarre dream where my underwear came to life and chased me. They were purple-and-white polka-dotted and had huge feet. Yes, feet. It was a dream. Dreams are always weird. Anyway, I ran and ran and ran but couldn't outrun my undies, so when I suddenly came upon a refrigerator, I ran inside and slammed the door shut tight. It was dark and scary, and, of course, exactly where my giant undies happened to be. I screamed, and they closed in on me, and then I woke up. I promptly threw away all my underwear that was either purple or polka-dotted, and never bought any that color ever again. Better safe than sorry.

I try to stay calm. I try not to think of polka dots. Or underwear. Or the color purple. I circle around a few times, hoping my eyeballs will adjust, but they don't cooperate. It's blacker than black. I'm grateful Clea and Nacho are here with me because there's no way giant undies could take all three of us.

"I'll get the door," I say, trying to sound plucky.

I palm the cold wall, but can't seem to find the handle. I frantically search every inch from top to bottom. My fingers start to go numb.

"Is everything all right?" I hear Clea ask. Or I think it's Clea. She sounds different. Like maybe she's being smothered by a giant pair of purple, polka-dotted undies?!

I have to get this door open!

"It's not here!" I yell. "The handle! It's not here!"

I'm convinced my nightmare is coming to life when WHOOSH the door opens and light floods the fridge. I'm blinded for a moment, but when my eyes adjust I see Nacho standing a few feet away from me, holding the door open. His head is cocked to one side.

"You are okay?"

I laugh and feel my cheeks go a little pink. "Yep. Just not a big fan of being trapped inside a dark refrigerator." I won't go into details about the undies. Some things are better left unsaid.

"I don't think anyone is," Clea agrees, and gives me a small smile, which makes me feel a little less embarrassed.

I appoint myself doorman, so we're not plunged into darkness again, while they grab the rest of the ingredients. Once we've collected everything, I close the fridge and follow them up to the workstation. I've barely set down the butter when

Tiffany strolls up and laces her arm through Nacho's.

"This class is really beneath me," she says as she pulls him to the other end of the workstation. "Did you know I'm an advanced chef? I can cook circles around these morons. I'm only here as a favor to my parents."

I grin at Clea. "Dude, my parents would be so proud. I'm finally a moron."

Clea tries not to laugh, but she can't help it and we both break out giggling as Tiffany looks down her nose at us.

It really is the most wonderful time of the year.

CHAPTER 5

Burn, Pancakes, Burn

P apa Shortdough claps his hands. "Okay, gang. Now that we've assembled our ingredients, it's time to get started."

I feel a little bubble of nervous excitement.

Papa nods at me. "Poppie and Clea you make the pancakes. Kale and Nacho, the burritos. Li and Tiffany, the oats. If you all start now, everything should finish around the same time, and then we get to eat your creations. Please clean your hands before you get started. Nick and I will roam around if you have questions."

After washing up, Clea and I take a minute to read through our recipe. We're making *Fluffy Pancakes with Fresh Berries*. I'm happy Papa put us together. Working with Tiffany probably would have sent me running to the door.

"I'll start by washing the fruit," I offer. "Do you want to start making the batter?"

Clea nods. "Sounds good."

I take the pudgy raspberries and plump blueberries over to the sink. I'm just about to dump raspberries into a colander when Papa taps my shoulder.

"Remember, raspberries are very delicate. It's best to gently place them in a bowl, cover them with water, and swirl the dirt away."

"What about blueberries?" I ask.

"They're usually pretty tough. Toss them in the colander, and shake away."

I wash all the berries as he suggested and take them back to the workstation. Clea is dumping yogurt into a large bowl.

"What's next?" I ask.

"Two cups of flour." She points to an enormous bag of flour that's at least five times as big as a normal bag. "It's really heavy."

I set the berries on the counter. "I'll help you. We can dump it into the measuring cup together."

"We never dump flour," Papa whispers from behind us. "We always spoon flour out of the bag like it's a delicate cloud."

I smile. "A cloud. I like that!"

He winks at me before moving a few feet down the workstation where Kale is chopping onions. "How's it going here?" he asks.

"Good. But my fingers already stink," Kale laughs. "I'm going to smell like onion all day."

Papa grins. "I have a great trick so you won't. When you're all finished chopping, rub your fingers on the steel faucet while washing your hands. It will take the onion smell right off your fingers."

Nacho is standing next to Kale, cracking eggs into a bowl. He wipes his eyes. "I hope it works because that smell is giving me crying."

Papa chuckles. "That is a strong onion." He pulls a pair of sunglasses out of his apron. "Here. Put this on. It will help block the fumes that are making your eyes water."

Nacho puts on the glasses. "Thanks. Now I see better what I'm doing," he laughs.

Papa hands him a whisk. "You can use this to really whip those eggs because that's what makes the scrambled eggs fluffy and light."

I'm loving all these little tips. Washing the berries.

Spooning out flour. How to avoid that onion smell. Look how much I've already learned and class just started. I'm starting to believe that maybe I can make Christmas Eve dinner after all.

Clea taps my shoulder and points to the bowl of batter. "The griddle is hot. Should we start cooking pancakes?"

Oh no. While I've been watching everyone else cook, she finished the recipe.

"Sorry, I got distracted," I apologize.

Her eyes widen. "Oh gosh no, don't be sorry. I only had to mix it together, and that was easy."

Now I feel even worse that I made her feel bad. "Well, thanks for finishing it. Let's go make some pancakes."

We walk a few feet to the back of the kitchen. Two, gleaming silver stoves sit side-by-side, connected by another smaller workstation. Each stove has four burners with a griddle in the middle.

Clea sets the batter on the workstation and stares at the griddle. "I'm a little nervous," she admits.

"Nothing to be nervous about," Papa says from behind us. Amazing how he seems to know just when he's needed. "It's just cooking!" He turns to me. "Poppie, I know you've made pancakes before, so why don't you cook the first few batches and then let Clea give it a whirl."

I nod, suddenly feeling proud that Papa thinks I know what I'm doing. I dip a small measuring cup into the batter, fill it up, and then pour it onto the hot griddle. The batter sputters and sizzles, and smells like rich, yeasty bread. My stomach grumbles.

"We don't have a plate to put them on," Clea suddenly exclaims, and rushes off.

While the pancakes cook, I look around to see how everyone else is doing. Nacho and Kale are cooking eggs at the other stove. Li is chopping apples. And our very own advanced chef, Tiffany, is bent over the metal workstation, using it as a mirror to apply her lipstick.

I see Nick waving at me from the other end of the workstation. Weird. He's suddenly acting very friendly. I wave back.

He shakes his head. "Poppie," he yells, "something's burning!"

I turn back to the griddle, and yelp. Smoke is steaming up from our pancakes! I grab the spatula, flip them over and groan.

They're black as night.

Burned.

Papa rushes over.

"Chef Burn strikes again," I mumble.

Papa shakes his head. "Not at all, Poppie. Your griddle was just too hot." He points to the knob on the front of the stove. "See. You have your flames set to HIGH."

Clea rushes over looking mortified. "I'm so sorry. I thought I turned it to MEDIUM when I pre-heated it."

Her cheeks are blazing red and tears spring to her eyes. Papa puts his arm around her and walks her a few steps away from the stove. I'm glad he's comforting her. He's really good at making people feel better.

I hate to see Clea so upset, but I'm honestly super relieved it wasn't my fault. I really think I can do this cooking thing. And lose twenty pounds! And get my first kiss! Things are looking up, dude!

I transfer the burned pancakes to the plate, and set them on the small workstation. I return to the stove, double check that the burner is on MEDIUM, and start scraping the burnt flecks off the griddle.

Papa taps my shoulder. "Your griddle is still too hot," he whispers in my ear, pointing to the control knobs that are back on HIGH again.

What?

"But I just checked them and they were on medium," I grumble.

He leans closer and whispers, "These stick out. You might have bumped into them and turned them higher. Try another batch, but don't lean against the stove this time." He pats me on the shoulder, and walks away.

I groan. So, it was my fault that the pancakes burned. I should have been watching them closer, and not looking around at what everyone else was doing. Maybe this is why I can't cook. Even when I follow the instructions, there are too many things that can go wrong. Things I can't plan ahead for, like the stupid stove changing temperatures just because I accidentally lean on it.

I hand Clea the pancake flipper. "Your turn."

She looks a little freaked out. "Um, I don't know."

"I do." I point to the other workstation where we made the batter. "As long as I stay over there you should be fine."

It takes a little coaxing, but I convince Clea that this is for the best. I stick around for moral support, but she doesn't really need me. She cooks the rest of the pancakes to a perfect, not-burnt, golden brown. She offers to trade a few times, but I feel like I'm doing an excellent job watching and I have no desire to burn anything, so I politely decline.

"Those look great," I gush as she adds the last pancake to our stack. "I really mean it. They look professional."

She blushes. "You really think so?"

I nod. "I think they look like Papa himself made them. Carry them up there with pride."

I follow her out of the kitchen with the bowl of mixed berries. At least, I didn't burn them.

The checkerboard counter has three notecards on it. We set the pancakes and berries in front of the card that reads *Fluffy Pancakes with Fresh Berries*. The other cards read *Cheesy Salsa Burritos* and *Cinnamon Oats and Apples*.

Nacho and Kale walk out of the kitchen. Nacho is carrying a platter of burritos.

He takes off Papa's shades and sets them on the counter, his eyes wide. "I am so hungry was hard not to eat all of this."

Kale nods. "I feel you, man. I hope we eat soon."

Li is right behind them, carrying a large bowl, followed by Tiffany and Papa.

"Okay, breakfast is served," Papa exclaims. "Everyone dig

in!"

Everyone loads up their plates. I'm super starving, but I don't want everyone to think I'm a pig so only I grab a little of everything before I sit down.

Kale sits on the stool next to me, tucks his tie into the neck of his t-shirt, and grins. "Pancakes look great, Poppie."

I gesture to Clea sitting next to me. "Tell Clea. She made them."

Kale has already shoveled in a huge bite so he gives her a thumbs up.

Clea blushes.

I take a bite of my pancake and groan with happiness. I can tell Clea didn't overmix them because the golden cake tastes light and fluffy. She's obviously a genius in the kitchen.

Papa claps his hands to get our attention. "While we're enjoying the fantastic breakfast you made, I want to chat about what we learned. Let's start with the pancakes." He gestures to Clea and me. "Great job, girls. They're really perfect. Because we live in the mountains at 8,700 feet, the recipe calls for more baking powder and less sugar to keep them fluffy. Then we add Greek yogurt for richness and extra protein."

"What did burning them add?" Tiffany pipes up, smirking at me.

Papa frowns.

But before he can respond, I blurt out, "Character."

I can fight my own battles. And I don't want anyone feeling sorry for me because I burn everything I cook. Only I can feel sorry for me.

I grin. "Yep. The burned ones add character." I widen my eyes and look straight at Tiffany when I add, "You may want to put a few more of those on your plate."

I hear Kale and Clea both choke on a chuckle.

"Now let's all be nice," Papa says, but I swear he's burying a smile. He Clears his throat. "Let's move on to the burritos. The secret to fluffy scrambled eggs is to really whisk them. Use those muscles and fluff them up. Salsa adds lots of flavor with few calories, and using all fresh ingredients to make the salsa is the key to its rich taste while also adding good vitamins. Nacho and Kale, great job on the burritos."

I mumble my approval because my mouth is full. Papa is right. The burritos are awesome! A soft tortilla filled with fluffy eggs and savory fresh tomatoes and onions is my new best friend. Sorry, Kale.

"Now let's move on to the oatmeal," Papa says. "I know it's rarely anyone's first choice, but made correctly it can be truly delicious. What does everyone think?"

"I'd eat this after a game," Li says, her snowman earrings dancing in agreement.

I tentatively take a bite. I can't remember the last time I had oatmeal and I don't think it was a good experience, but I'm pleasantly surprised. The oats are warm and cinnamony, like a fresh-out-of-the-oven oatmeal cookie. The fresh apple adds a tart crispness and the toasted walnuts give a rich crunch. These oats may be better than a cookie. Although no way am I saying that out loud. It might ruin my rep.

Papa smiles. "Eating this after a game or before you hit the slopes would be an excellent choice. It's high in fiber so you're not hungry ten minutes later. The walnuts provide protein and healthy fat. And the apples give it a natural sweetness. You did a great job, Li!"

I notice he didn't include Tiffany in his compliment, but she doesn't seem to care. She's barely touched any food on her plate, and is staring off into the kitchen.

"I'm very proud of this Yum Yum class," Papa gushes with pride. "Everything is really delicious."

He's right. The pancakes are tasty. The burritos are excellent. And the oatmeal is surprisingly yum. Who knew healthy could taste so good?

This has been a sweet class. I definitely feel more confident now. And with all these new healthy recipes, I just know I'm going to lose that twenty pounds.

And then I'll finally get my first kiss.

Maybe even under the Christmas tree.

CHAPTER 6

You Gotta Tweak the Plan

Once we're finished eating, everyone helps clean up the mess. Even Tiffany has to pitch in. She complains when Papa puts her on wash duty, until he asks her exactly what she cooked today, and that left her speechless.

Kale and I are the last ones to leave.

"That was a great class, Papa!" Kale gushes as he puts on his jacket.

"Glad you liked it!" Papa tilts his head. "What about you, Poppie?"

"I thought it was great, too. I can't wait to try making these recipes at home. I never knew healthy food could taste so good."

Kale thumps my arm. "Especially when it's not burned," he jokes, and then seeing my face quickly adds, "You made really good pancakes!"

I frown. "That's because Clea cooked them." I shake my head. "Who am I kidding? I'll never be able to make these at home. I burn everything. It's a curse. A plague upon me. A tumor on my soul." I know I'm being a little dramatic, but I don't care. I hang my head. "I'll never be able to cook."

Papa chuckles. "Just because you burned a couple pancakes doesn't mean you can't cook."

I nod. "Uh huh! I burn everything. I even made a plan and followed it, and I still burned the pancakes."

Kale arches an eyebrow. "You made a plan to cook pancakes?"

This shouldn't really surprise Kale. He knows I like to make plans. I like to know that things will go the way they should. That there will be no surprises.

I shrug. "Well it wasn't quite as elaborate as some of my other plans, but I figured that if I followed Papa's recipe exactly then I wouldn't burn anything."

Papa smiles. "Just because you make a plan doesn't mean it will work out exactly how you planned it."

My eyebrows shoot through the ceiling. "That's crazy talk! The whole point of making a plan is so everything does work out."

Papa sits on the stool next to me. "That could be why cooking may be a bit hard for you right now. Anybody can start with a plan, or in this case, a recipe, but a chef must also be willing to change the recipe if needed. A great chef has to be flexible. Maybe there are no blueberries. What can she use? How about strawberries? Maybe the cake fell flat. Make it into brownies instead." He smiles. "Tweaks in a recipe are sometimes how a new incredible food is discovered because a great chef is not afraid of changes." He leans closer. "I even changed one of my recipes this morning."

I sit up straighter. "You changed your cookies?"

He shakes his head. "No. I tweaked my coffee cake by throwing in a little chocolate, and guess what?"

I think I know the answer, but I humor him. "What?"

He spreads his arms wide. "Everyone is raving about how it tastes better than ever! I think the true secret to being a great chef is being willing to tweak your recipes." He winks. "Or your plan."

I'm not going to argue with him, but I'm pretty sure he's wrong. What's the point of a recipe if you don't follow it? And what's the point of a plan if you have to change it? But I accept that we're going to disagree, so I change the subject.

"Speaking of your cookies, didn't you have a secret about them that you were going to tell us?"

Papa's eyes crinkle as he chuckles. "Nice try, Poppie, but if I told you, then it wouldn't be a secret anymore." He stands up, grabs a towel off the counter and throws it over his shoulder. "Now I better get back to work. I'll see you two for class tomorrow." He winks. "We're going to have a contest."

"To figure out your secret?"

He shakes his head. "Nope. See you tomorrow."

I watch him disappear back into the kitchen, whistling a happy tune. This secret is making him very happy, and I love seeing him happy, but it's a secret and I just have to know what it is.

I look at Kale and nod. "We're going to figure out his secret."

Kale stands up and shakes his head. "Pass."

He starts walking towards the door, so I pull on my jacket, and catch up to him near the front.

"We have to," I beg.

"No."

"But I have a plan."

Kale stops in front of the revolving door, turns around, and laughs. "Poppie, you always have a plan."

I waggle my eyebrows and give him my biggest grin. "You know me so well." I step into the revolving door, but only circle a few times before popping out onto the snowy sidewalk. My world-record will have to wait. I have other things on my plate now.

Kale and I turn left and start walking down Main Street. I inhale a long, deep breath of cold air that makes me feel like I've just eaten a peppermint. The clock at The Rock bongs twice to announce two o'clock. A bear carved out of beetle-kill wood totters out of a hole in the center of the clock, roars, and then disappears back into the hole. It's mid-afternoon but the winter sun has already set behind the mountain and shadows are creeping up the storefronts. It will be pitch dark by four.

We pass The Slope Bookstore. The front window is draped with silver garland and my favorite book, *The Night Before Christmas in Ski Country,* is propped up on a present wrapped in shiny red paper. Usually I'd stop in to see what's new, but all I can think about is Papa's secret.

I nudge Kale's shoulder. "Come on, you know you want to help me."

He rolls his eyes and doesn't answer. He thinks I snoop too much. I call it being informed. He calls it meddling.

"Don't you want to know his secret?" I ask.

"Nope, couldn't care less."

"Even if it has something to do with *Yum Yum?*"

That gets his attention. "What do you mean?"

Now that I have him hooked, I don't answer. Kale often needs time to let his imagination go wild before he agrees to help me with a plan. I skip ahead to the stoplight and push the crosswalk button.

Kale hurries to catch up with me. "You think his secret has something to do with the contest tomorrow?"

The contest? My shoulders slump. I had forgotten about the contest. And unless it's a contest to see can burn food the fastest, I'm bound to lose.

And I hate losing.

I slap my forehead. "Oh geez, I totally forgot. I don't think I'm going to make it for the contest tomorrow. I have an important meeting in... Morocco."

Kale laughs. "Right." He raises one dark eyebrow. "If you don't go back, you may never find out Papa's secret."

I groan. Unfortunately, Kale knows me as well as I know him. I don't want to go back to class without knowing what the contest is about because I can't make a plan to win if I don't know what I'm winning, but I also need to go back to the market to find out what secret Papa is hiding. Whew.

"Okay, okay." I wave my hand. "I'll reschedule my meeting. I only hope the lovely people of Morocco will forgive me."

The WALK flashes, and Kale starts running.

"Race you across!" he yells over his shoulder. "Loser buys the cookies tomorrow."

I sprint after him. "Cheater!" I yell, but I don't really mean it. I would have done the exact same thing.

Kale reaches the other side first and fist punches the air. "The winnah!" He points to himself while jumping up and down, his tie flapping around like a streamer, looking super ridiculous. Which, of course, makes me bust out laughing.

"You're a total goof." I manage to sputter.

"Maybe," he admits. "But this goof is going to have two cookies tomorrow," he waggles two fingers in front of my face, "since you're buying."

I high five his fingers. "You got it, goof."

We walk a little farther down the street into what here in Butte we call a neighborhood. Each family's property is a few acres surrounded by forests of towering evergreens, so it's a little different than what you may find in a city. Most people only see trees out their windows, not their neighbor washing dishes next door.

We stop at the cross-rail fence surrounding the mini-ranch owned by Miss Sweettarte, an older lady who moved here from Texas a couple years ago. The pasture is white with snow and dotted with horses. There's a black-and-white paint named Takoda, a white horse with a cloud-shaped, brown splotch named Sky, and a brother-sister pair of brown mustangs named Cat and Dog. Right now they all look like big teddy bears in their shaggy, winter coats. Miss Sweettarte told me she may have rescued them from being dog food, but they all rescued her right back. I'm not quite certain what she means by that, but it sounded like a good thing.

We spot Miss Sweettarte at the end of her driveway, sitting on her pony, looking our way.

I wave to her.

She waves back and trots up to meet us, posting so perfectly that the tips of her gray hair hanging out from under her helmet don't move at all. Miss Sweettarte is short and stick thin but makes me think of warm apple pie. My mom once said that she's sweet as sugar and southern as chicken fried steak, and I would definitely agree.

She stops crisply in front of us. "Good afternoon, y'all," she sings in her Southern drawl.

"Good afternoon," Kale and I answer almost perfectly in sync. We try to be polite and use good manners with Miss Sweettarte, mostly because she doesn't allow us not to.

I take my glove off and reach my hand under her pony's nose. "Hi, Astra," I murmur.

Astra snorts softly and nuzzles my hand. Her lips nibble my palm, leaving a silky trail of slobber as she searches for food.

I laugh. "No treats today, girl."

Miss Sweettarte backs Astra up a few steps. "Any chance you just came from Papa's Market?" she asks with a chuckle.

I nod. "Yes, ma'am."

Yes. I said ma'am. I am *very* polite with Miss Sweettarte.

"That explains her behavior," Miss Sweettarte says, drawing her pink-lipsticked mouth up into a huge grin. She runs her hand through Astra's mane. "This girl can smell his cookies from a mile away. They're her favorite treat." She shakes her head. "Used to be carrots until that handsome devil spoiled her." Miss Sweettarte pretends to fan herself. "So handsome."

I almost laugh out loud, but I stop myself. Miss Sweettarte is as old as my grandma and she thinks Papa Shortdough is handsome? I knew they were dating, but the way she's smiling she must really, *really* like him. Interesting. I wonder if he knows.

"Where's Old Gray?" Kale asks, nodding at the horses in the pasture.

Miss Sweettarte tsks. "He's in the stall. That old rascal cut his leg this morning."

A thick line forms between Kale's eyebrows. "Is he okay?"

Kale has a soft spot for Old Gray. When Miss Sweettarte rescued him last year, he was really sick and really skinny. Kale helped nurse him back to health. He even spent a few nights sitting outside his stall. That lucky horse went from looking like a skeleton to a pudgy, abominable snow horse.

Miss Sweettarte waves her hand. "Gracious, yes! He's just mad as a mule chasing bumblebees that I locked him up." She smiles at Kale. "Don't you worry. He's been through so much in his 30 years that I don't think an itty bitty cut is going to slow him down."

Kale nods. "Well, you know I'm happy to help if he needs anything."

Miss Sweettarte opens her mouth to say something but her words are drowned out by window-rattling music. A mud-splattered, red 4x4 truck screeches to a stop right in front of us. Astra trots in place, jerking her head anxiously. As Miss Sweettarte turns her in a circle to calm her, the passenger door opens and guess who steps out of the truck?

Nick.

Joy to the world.

Or not.

CHAPTER 7

Cheesy Puffs and Cookies

Nick steps out of the truck, slams the door and walks past all of us as if we're invisible. Maybe because he's wearing all black, he thinks he's a ninja and we can't see him.

"Nick," Miss Sweettarte sings out.

He turns around. "Yes?"

She motions to us. "Have you met my darlin' next-door neighbors, Poppie and Kale?"

Nick sighs. "Yes, NaMiss But I can't hang with the little kids now cause I got stuff to do." And without another word, he turns and walks up the driveway towards Miss Sweettarte's house.

Little kids? Nams?

Miss Sweettarte frowns as she watches Nick walk away, but when she turns back to us, she's smiling again. "I'm tickled y'all already met. Nick is my grandson."

I almost choke.

"He just moved in with me, and will be a sophomore at Butte High School when Christmas break is over." Her eyes crinkle a little. "I promise he's really sweet as a peach once you get to know him. And I know he's a year older than y'all, but hopefully y'all can all hang out and become good friends."

I almost snort out loud. Chances of me becoming friends with Nick would be right about when pigs fly and open drive-throughs in the sky that serve bacon cheeseburgers.

Miss Sweettarte pats her pony's neck. "Well, I best get these big sweeties fed. Ta ta, darlings!" She sings as she wiggles her fingers in a wave before trotting away.

I wait until she's out of earshot before I freak out.

"Nick is her grandson? Seriously?!" I exhale a huge sigh. "I bet his last name is I-am-definitely-*not*-a-Sweettarte."

Kale snorts. "Probably. But us *little kids* may never know."

I shake my head. "Yeah. He's a big, bad sophomore, and we're just lowly freshman."

"Lowly, *little* freshman." Kale laughs. "You're six feet tall, and I'm six-one. It's kind of fun that someone thinks we're little."

I giggle. Kale's right. And little is definitely better than huge.

We walk a few more minutes until we reach the end of Miss Sweettarte's mini-ranch and the beginning of the driveway I share with Kale. My house is next to Miss Sweettarte, and Kale's house is next to mine. Our houses share the lower part of the driveway, but are separated by over an acre of trees. My driveway disappears to the left around a big grove of aspens and Kale's driveway veers to the right through a bunch of evergreens.

I grab the mail out of my box. "Want to come over?"

He shakes his head. "Can't. Mom's coming home early and taking me Christmas shopping."

"Oh goodie! Call me later to let me know what you bought me."

"Will do," he laughs. "Later."

He heads towards his house, and I start the walk up to mine. My driveway faces west so it's still bathed in the fading sunshine. The bare aspens look like thin, pale ghosts as I walk past them, but I know they're not dead. They're happy and waiting to burst with life when spring rolls around again, and they always welcome me home.

I reach the top of my drive and stop, gasping for breath. I know I just walked straight uphill but it was only a quarter mile. Am I that out of shape? I never get this tired snowboarding. I'm about to head inside and watch a movie when I remember something Kale's mom said. She's a well-known dietitian, and I overheard her saying something about "you have to move to lose." And if I want to lose twenty pounds and get my first kiss, vegging on the couch isn't going to get me there.

I take my big thighs down and back up my driveway one more time. I'm aiming for a mile but my lungs are burning and my legs are wobbling so I figure three-quarters is good. Maybe I can do a mile tomorrow.

I punch the code into the garage door and wait while it opens. I love my house. It's surrounded by evergreen trees, has a huge wraparound porch, and it's really colorful. The front door and garage doors are red, and the siding and roof are green. I walk into the garage, open the door leading into the laundry room, and I'm immediately knocked to the ground as one hundred pounds of white-fluffy-love pounces on me.

"Hi, Lucy Lu," I croon to our dog as she settles herself onto my lap. She's huge like me, but I don't tell her because she thinks she's a tiny puppy.

I scratch her ears and neck, and she rewards me with lots of slobbery kisses. We rescued her from the pound a few years ago and I'm pretty sure she believes slobbery kisses every day are the best way to thank us.

I stand up and try to brush the gobs of white hair off my jeans. "Come on, girl. Let's get you a treat."

Lucy's tail shoots straight into the air. She knows that word as well as I do. We both adore treats.

Our kitchen is colorful, too. The cabinets are white, but the barstools are purple, the appliances are red, and Lucy's dog treats are in a jar shaped like a fat, yellow chicken.

I lift the chicken head, grab a bacon treat for Lucy, and toss it into the air. She jumps up, snatches it before it reaches the ground, and trots off to the next room with her prize.

I pour myself a glass of water and sit down on a barstool. It's not even three o'clock. I still have a couple hours before my brother and parents get home. I don't have any homework because it's break. I don't feel like putting my clean clothes away. I already wrapped my Christmas presents. What should I do?

Then I remember the contest Papa Shortdough mentioned. I groan. I bet it's a cooking contest. My stomach tightens. There's no way I'll win.

Unless it's a race to see who can burn something the fastest.

I glare at the oven. "It's all your fault, you know. I like to cook and I could be great at it. You obviously like to cook or you wouldn't be in this profession. You'd be a sink, or a fridge." I sigh. "I wish we could learn to work together. We could be a great team and create a famous recipe that changes the world." I stand up and stare into the middle distance. "I can see it now. Me as a world-renowned chef," I glance down at the oven, "twenty pounds lighter, of course." I stare back into my dream. "I will travel all over the globe teaching people how to make my secret recipe. Everyone will come together to cook and eat my secret recipe, and that will finally bring peace to the world."

I glance at the oven to see what it thinks of my amazing plan. No reaction. I shrug. Not everyone can be a visionary. But I know what I have to do. I'll make something deliciously mind-blowing and bring it to *Yum Yum* tomorrow. Everyone will rave about how good it is, and beg that I share it with the world. Then it won't matter if I lose the contest because they'll all be thinking about how delicious my secret recipe is. It's a perfect plan.

But what to make? It has to be something everyone loves. And something memorable. Like Papa's cookies.

That's it! I'll make cookies. Everyone loves cookies!

I toss back the rest of my water, slip my thumbs into my jean belt loops, and swagger over to the oven. "There's only room for one chef in this kitchen," I drawl. I punch the BAKE button with authority. "And it's going to be me."

The oven doesn't argue or explode, so I decide that's a good sign. I pull out my mom's chocolate-chip cookie recipe, and grin with happy memories. The notecard is tattered and stained, but still readable. She made these cookies for me and my brother every Monday when we were in grade school. They were chock full of chocolate chips and pecans, but the best part was that she'd always write what she loved about me on a napkin that was wrapped around the cookie.

Chocolate Chip Love Cookies. It's a perfect name.

I collect all my ingredients, and follow her recipe exactly, paying special attention to all her scribbled notes. When it's all mixed together, I taste the dough. Yum! Just as good as I remember. But I need to make them my recipe. My secret recipe. I need to add something that makes them incredible enough to save the world.

I search the cabinet. Oats. Too expected. Cereal. Nah. Pasta. Weird. Then I see them. Cheesy puffs. Yes. I love cheesy puffs. My dad says they turn me into a magician because every time I have a bag in my hand, they all disappear. This has to be my secret, special ingredient. It was meant to be.

I wrestle the bag open and taste a few. That airy crunch and artificial orange flavoring will be perfect. Cheesy puffs in cookies! I'm a genius.

I remind myself that eating the whole bag of cheesy puffs will not bring me closer to my first kiss, so I add a handful to the bowl and stuff the bag back into the cabinet. I mix the puffs into the dough, admiring how the orange coloring swirls throughout the dough like shooting stars in a cheesy galaxy. I plop huge chunks of dough onto a tray and shove it into the oven.

This is a sweet plan. My cookies are bound to be as popular as *Papa's Triple-Chocolate Cookies*. And won't Mom be surprised to see that I made cookies for her this time? I grab my cell. I have to tell Kale about my new creation.

He answers my video call immediately. "What's up?" His face pops into the screen, and I can see he's in his room.

"You back from shopping?"

He nods. "And don't try to guess your present."

"Okay."

"Okay? Just like that? Poppie what's going on? *You* don't want to figure out a secret?"

I wave my hand. "Oh, don't worry, I will. But later. I need to tell you something first. Guess what I'm doing?" I aim the video so he can see the mess on the counter.

His eyebrows go up. "You're cooking?"

I nod. "Yes! And I've just created a cookie that is guaranteed to bring peace and harmony to the world and make me famous, and you can say you knew me way back when."

"Cool. What kind of cookie?"

"Well, I started with my mom's recipe, but then guess what I added?"

"What?"

"Cheesy puffs!"

I see his nose wrinkle. He doesn't say anything.

"Well?"

He chuckles. "How'd they turn out?"

I shrug. "I don't know yet. They're still baking."

I look over at the oven. Smoke is curling around it in a grin.

Maybe it's not the most wonderful time of the year.

CHAPTER 8

My Parents Are So Weird

I toss my phone onto the counter. "Hold on a minute!" I yell to Kale.

I grab potholders, yank the tray out of the oven, and set it on the counter. I'm hoping something else was burning in the oven and causing all the smoke, but as I examine the cookies I want to scream.

I burned them.

To a crisp.

Again.

I poke a cookie with my finger and it sighs a wisp of smoke. I glare at the oven and swear I can hear it laughing.

I pick up my cell. "Well…, they're a bit dark."

"How dark?" Kale asks.

I frown into the camera.

"That bad?"

I nod.

"Well, at least you tried."

I sigh. "But I burned something AGAIN." I shake my head. "That's it. The oven is definitely out to get me. I'm done with cooking. I'm giving it up. The oven wins. I'll never be a chef."

"Don't say that," Kale pleads. "So, you burned the cookies.

That doesn't mean you'll never be a chef. I mean, look what you learned in class today."

I snort. "Yeah. I learned how to burn pancakes."

Kale laughs. "Well, yes. But we also learned how to make healthy breakfasts. And weren't they better than your bag of chalky donuts?"

I shrug. "Eh."

He narrows his eyes. "Eh?"

"Fine. Yes. They were good. And I know if I want to lose twenty pounds to get my first kiss, I need to cut back on the donuts."

He frowns. "That's not what I'm saying."

I wave my hand. "I know. But I gotta go. I need to get rid of this mess before everyone comes home."

"Ok." He winks at me. "Later, great Chef Burn."

I roll my eyes. "Ha ha, very funny."

"Seriously, don't worry about it. OK?"

I shrug. "Ok."

He grins. "Well, I know you're lying, but call me if you want to talk more."

I nod, and end our call.

Chef Burn. That's me. I guess I should be happy that at least I'm the chef of something.

I set my phone back down on the counter, and reach out to grab the tray, totally blanking that it was just in a very hot oven. I shriek and yank my sizzling fingers away, sending the tray flying across the room and flinging the cookie black holes through space until they shatter all over the white tile floor.

Yep. The oven is definitely laughing at me now.

Lucy races into the kitchen and starts scarfing up the burnt pieces. I know chocolate is really bad for dogs so I've just grabbed her collar when she immediately gags and spits out every piece she inhaled. She hacks for a few minutes and then looks up at me with her amber eyes, looking very displeased with my choice of treat.

I hold out my hands. "Hey, I didn't tell you to eat them."

She sniffs with displeasure and walks out of the kitchen.

I grab the small broom and dustpan from under the sink and start relocating my failed experiment to the trash. I put away all the ingredients, wash the dishes, and wipe everything down. Soon the kitchen is back to normal and I'm pretty sure no one will suspect I was cooking. I sniff the air. Ick. But they will definitely suspect I was burning something.

I crack the window open above the sink. I'm waving in the cool air and pushing the burnt smell out when I hear my brother, Berg, come in the garage door.

Uh oh.

I slam the window shut, tie up the trash bag of evidence, and hide it behind me just as he walks into the kitchen. He tosses his keys on the counter and sets down two pizza boxes.

"Yo, Sis. What's up?"

Berg's two years older than me, half a foot taller, and doesn't cook either. If our parents are working late, he brings home dinner after whatever extreme sport he's dominating. Right now he's crushing downhill ski racing. Lots of speed and major sick crashes. And helmet head.

Except for Berg. He never has helmet head. We share the same blond hair, but while mine looks like I've been electrocuted, his always looks like he just stepped out of a surfboard commercial.

I smile and lean against the counter, trying to act all casual. "Not much going on here. Same old, same old. How was racing today?"

"Oh, man, it was unreal!" Berg starts. "Dean took this run…" He stops mid-sentence and sniffs the air. His eyebrows go up. "What's that smell?"

I try to look all innocent. "Smell? What smell?" I nod toward the pizza boxes, desperately hoping warm cheese and savory sausage will cover up the smell of scorched cheesy puffs. "I only smell pizza." I inhale a long whiff. "Yum. So, what about Dean?"

Berg chuckles. "Nice try. I'm not buying it. What'd you

burn this time?"

I sigh. I'm a terrible liar so I don't even try. Plus, Berg's pretty cool.

I hold up the trash bag. "Cookies." I frown. "But they would have been sweet if our oven wasn't evil and out to get me."

Berg coughs. "You must have really fried them because it reeks in here." He motions towards the window. "You might want to open that before Mom and Dad get home."

I set down the trash bag and open the window. "I had it open before you came home, but I guess it didn't help." If he thought the kitchen smelled bad now, he should have been here half an hour ago.

He grins. "At least you didn't burn down the house again."

I roll my eyes. "Dude, I never burned down the house."

When I was four-years-old and my parents were still sleeping at the late hour of 3:30 a.m, I decided to make my own breakfast. I'd seen my mom do it a million times, so how hard could it be? I dumped a packet of oatmeal into a bowl, put it in the microwave, closed the door, pushed some buttons, and sat down to wait. I forgot to add milk, and microwaving dried oatmeal for ten minutes tends to make it smoke. A lot.

Contrary to what everyone says, I didn't burn down the house. I only set off the smoke alarms. No one talks about how independent I was cooking breakfast at such a young age, they only remember the fire trucks. All three of them.

I'm about to remind Berg of how self-sufficient I was when I hear the garage door open.

"That would be Mom and Dad," Berg says.

I slam the window shut, grab the trash bag and fling it behind me. "Please don't say anything."

Berg makes a zipping motion across his lips, and winks.

Mom and Dad walk into the kitchen together, both of them grinning ear-to-ear. They're both wearing head-to-toe black leather, and their previously white-blond hair is blacker than my cookies. I'm speechless.

For as long as I can remember, my parents have been hippies. I mean, real 1970s flower children. Mom always wears her long, flowy, blond hair over a long, flowy, flower dress, and Dad always ties his long, blond, curly hair into a low ponytail and wears a concert t-shirt. I've never seen them wear anything else.

Until today.

Mom giggles. "What do you think?"

"You cut your hair." I manage to blurt out.

Mom pats her midnight bob and giggles like the five-year old down the street. "Nah. I just tucked it under. Do you like it?"

I don't know what to say. I think I'm in shock.

Berg pipes up. "I think it's rad."

Dad flips his dark ponytail over his back. "Groovy! We thought a new look would help us fit in better at our new school."

I almost drop the trash bag. "New school?"

Dad grins so wide I can see where he lost his tooth when he and Mom went rappelling for his fortieth birthday. He beams at Mom. "You tell them, Lamikins."

Mom jumps up and down, her ebony bob fanning out like a parachute. "We're going to become private investigators!"

I burst out laughing. They're totally messing with us. Mom and Dad are the world's purest hippies. They own a flower shop, wear sandals with socks (even in the winter!), and preach karma and unicorns and peace to everyone. Our parents as down and dirty PI's? That's a good one.

Dad cocks his head. "We're not joking."

I stop laughing. "Huh?" I hiccup.

Mom digs around in her floppy purse and pulls out a glossy brochure. She holds it at arm's length and squints to read it without her glasses. "The Expert School of Private Investigation. Where anyone can learn how to set your inner snoop free." She's beaming when she looks up at us. "Doesn't that sound cool?"

I nod slowly. Sounds cool to me. But to my parents? It sounds like they have lost their minds.

Dad sniffs the air. "Did someone burn the pizza?"

Berg shakes his head. "Nope."

I grit my teeth, waiting to be accused, but luckily Lucy trots into the kitchen and comes to my rescue. She runs to greet my parents, takes in their new look, and starts to growl.

Mom laughs. "Lucy! It's just me."

The minute she hears Mom's voice, Lucy's tail starts wagging. She tilts her head to one side and woofs, probably asking "What the heck did you do to yourself?" Mom reaches down to scratch her, and Lucy rolls over and out lolls her tongue.

Dad sniffs the air again. "If someone didn't burn the pizza, then what's that smell?"

He's looking directly at me and I'm pretty sure I'm toast-burnt toast- but Berg saves me.

"I'm starved." Berg grabs the pizza and heads towards the dining room. "Let's eat and you can tell us more about this new gig you got going on."

"I am surprisingly famished," Mom admits. As she follows Dad and Berg into the dining room, I hear her ask, "Wonder if being a private investigator gives you a bigger appetite?"

I race out to the garage, bury the evidence deep in the garbage can, and rush back to the dining room just as everyone is sitting down.

Our dining room is as colorful as the rest of our house. Dad found an old Ping-Pong table in someone's trash years ago. Mom repainted it bright green and added white daisies. On one side there's a pink-and-yellow plaid couch that burps stuffing whenever anyone sits on it, and on the other side are an assortment of plastic lawn chairs in various shades of red and green.

I sit in my favorite, fire-engine red chair, grab a piece of pizza, and plop it onto my plate. I take a bite, and gooey, warm cheese coats my tongue. I take another bite and try to chew slower. I know eating an entire pie is definitely not on my first kiss diet.

"When do you start PI school?" Berg asks, stuffing half a piece into his mouth. He's not huge, and probably never will be, and he can eat an entire pie.

"Tomorrow," Dad says.

I choke on my pizza. "Tomorrow?

Mom nods. "If we want to get connected with our inner busybodies, we must start as soon as possible." She explains this as if she's telling me about a new flower she brought in from a small, organic farm in Idaho instead of how she's going to learn to snoop and eavesdrop and nark on unsuspecting people.

"And you're starting tomorrow?" I ask again, thinking I must have heard wrong because they surely won't start a new school on the day before Christmas Eve.

"Yeah! Far out, right?" Dad gushes. "We're going to learn to operate surveillance equipment, the best ways to spot evidence, and how to hypnotize."

I shake my head. "Hypnotize?"

Mom claps her hands together. "Yes! So we can get more info out of the perps." She looks at Dad. "Did I say that right, babe?"

He nods. "I think so."

Mom looks back at me. "And do you know what the best part is? All the teachers are private investigators working in the field!" She wipes sauce off Dad's cheek, and shivers. "I can't believe we not only get to meet them, but learn from them!"

I have no response. I'm utterly dumbfounded. I feel like I'm in the middle of some freaky movie where aliens take over the parents' bodies and turn them into lunatics.

"What about *The Right Stem*?" I ask. "You're not going to close it are you?"

Mom shakes her head. "Oh, golly no! We will still run our flower shop during the day. The PI school is at night, so we'll drive down the hill to the school after we close up."

"Like after our family dinner?"

Even though we eat take-out and microwavable meals, I love our family dinners. We talk. We act silly. We laugh. I look forward to our time together.

Mom shakes her head. "No, I'm sorry, Poppie. We probably won't be home for dinner most nights."

I sigh. Well that bites.

Looks like I'll be having a blue Christmas after all.

CHAPTER 9

Why Do I Even Try?

Berg is about to inhale his eighth piece of pizza. "Why do you want to be private investigators?"

Dad grins. "Can't tell you."

I raise an eyebrow. "Why not?"

He grins even wider as he leans close and whispers. "Because it's a secret."

Both of my eyebrows shoot through my head and land on the ceiling. My parents have a secret! Papa has a secret! Everyone has secrets!

I throw my last piece of pizza back onto my plate. "Seriously?" I screech. I debate flinging myself on the floor and throwing a major tantrum until I remind myself that I'm almost fifteen, not two. "It's a secret, and you can't even tell your own children?"

Dad shakes his head. "Nope. Sorry, Poppie Pop. No can do." He smiles and takes another bite of pizza. "So, how was your day? Didn't you have your first cooking class?"

I frown. I know what he's trying to do. He's changing the subject. I'm a pro at it. I do it all the time when I don't want to talk about something. Well, you know what? I'm going to change the subject, too. Because if they won't tell me their secret then I'm not going to tell them anything about my day.

I stand up and start stacking plates. "Thanks for grabbing pizza, Berg." I force happiness into my voice. "Can we try that new Indian restaurant tomorrow?" See. I know how to change the subject, too.

"Sounds good," Berg says. He glances over at Mom and Dad. "You guys okay with that?"

Mom hands me her plate. "Get whatever sounds good to the two of you. We have a late delivery tomorrow so Dad and I will grab something on the way to school."

A horrible thought enters my mind. "Will you be here for Christmas Eve dinner?"

Mom frowns. "We don't know yet."

I feel my temper explode, like the time I turned on a blender full of fruit and yogurt and forgot to put on the lid. Smoothie everywhere!

I slam the plates so hard onto the table that I'm lucky they don't break. "Well, that's just fabulous." I pace back and forth, waving my arms around. "That's Christmas Eve, you know? Christmas Eve!" My voice rises. "As in the special night before Christmas that I planned on making us all a special dinner? As in the reason I'm taking this cooking class that now has some sort of secret contest that I can't plan for so I can't win." I shriek, throwing my arms in the air. "And there's another secret!"

I pause my ranting to catch my breath and notice everyone is staring at me. Mouths open. Eyes wide. Ready to calm me with herbal tea, or worse, a soothing meditative chant. Oops. Better dial back the frenzy.

I exhale. "Sorry about that."

I pick up the plates and hurry into the kitchen. Mom follows me. She takes the plates from me, sets them on the counter and wraps me in a hug. Luckily, there's no chanting.

"I'm sorry, Poppie Pop," she murmurs. "We're all really proud of you for taking this cooking class and wanting to make us dinner." She releases me from the hug and brushes a stray hair away from my cheek. "I know how much you like to plan ahead, so I promise I'll find out more tomorrow, and we will try our absolute best to be here for your Christmas Eve dinner."

I don't say anything.

"Okay?" she asks.

I want to tell her no. That it's not okay. I want to ask her why she has to change things? Why does she have to go to school? Why does she have to miss my dinner?

But I don't say any of those things. It's okay. Really. I'm not taking the cooking class to cook for them anyway. Who cares about family dinners. All I care about is losing twenty pounds so I can finally get my first kiss.

I force a smile and nod. "Okay."

Mom squeezes me in another hug. "Are you really okay?"

I'm not feeling particularly jolly, but I know that's not what she wants to hear. "Sure. I'm all good. Thanks, Mom. You go relax. It's my turn to clean up."

I don't think she believes me, but she hugs me once more before joining Dad on the couch in the living room. I hear them laughing at something on TV as I load the dishwasher. I know it's selfish, but I don't want to hear any more about their PI school so instead of joining them when I'm finished, I head upstairs to Berg's room.

I knock on his open door.

He looks up from a skiing magazine he's reading. "Hey, what's up?"

I like Berg's room. The walls are a deep blue, and everything is always neat, organized and tidy. Just like Berg.

I walk over to his crisply-made bed, and plop down next to him. "I think our parents are loony."

Berg snorts. "Snoops, too, apparently."

"Guess we won't be seeing them much." I try to sound like I don't care.

"Maybe," he says. "But at least they're living their dream. They always said that if we want something we're the only ones who can make it happen." He grins. "You have to admit, it's kind of cool to see them take their own advice."

I roll my eyes. I hate it when what he says makes way more sense than whatever I'm whining about.

I shrug. "Yeah, I guess."

He returns to his magazine so I figure I should go. I stand up and walk to the door.

"Poppie?"

I turn back around. "Yeah?"

"You all right?"

That's my big brother. Always looking out for me.

I nod. "Yep. Thanks."

I walk across the hall to my room, which is the total opposite of Berg's. I may be an excellent planner, but I'm the farthest thing from organized. I have papers lying everywhere, a million stuffed animals loafing on my bed, and clothes smothering my floor. But it's my room, and I love it.

I close my door, shuffle through last week's dirty clothes, and flop onto my bed. My phone barks at me. It's Kale texting me.

Meet @mailboxes 9:30 -walk to class?

Ugh. Don't remind me. I change the subject.

Parents want 2B snoops!

What?!

My words exactly.

Do they know it's Christmastime at all?

CHAPTER 10

Amazingly, I Don't Burn Lunch

Kale shakes his head as we walk down Main Street towards Papa's Market. "I just can't picture your parents as private investigators." He chuckles. "I mean, your mom wears mumus."

I sigh. "Not anymore. Black leather head to toe." Huge, fluffy snowflakes are falling around us, and I catch one on my tongue and pretend it's ice cream.

Kale raises his eyebrows. "Black leather? For real?"

I groan. "Yes."

"Your dad?"

"Same."

He laughs out loud. "*That* I have to see."

"Oh, I'm sure you will," I roll my eyes. "It's obviously their new uniform or something."

Kale flings an arm over my shoulder. "Oh, come on, Poppie. It's not that bad. Maybe it's just a phase. Like that time they added that herbal powder to everything you ate."

I make a face. "Ugh! That stuff was disgusting." I raise one eyebrow, wondering if he remembers. "Especially on fries."

Kale shakes his head. "Don't remind me! Man! I had to bathe my tongue in yogurt for a month to get that taste out of my mouth."

That makes me laugh. "Yeah, sorry about that. I just wanted you to share the experience."

He snorts. "Next time keep it to yourself."

We walk a few minutes in silence. With Christmas Eve only a day away, the ski resort is busy with holiday visitors. I step around a man taking a photo of the resort's clock, then fall back into step with Kale.

"If this is just another phase, then why not tell me the reason they want to become private investigators?" I ask him. "The herbal thing was because the flu was really bad that year. But why exactly does one sign up to become a PI? Are their flowers misbehaving? Is there an evil flower shop in the next town that's stealing their business? And why is it a secret? I mean, come on, just tell me why." A feathery snowflake attaches to my eyelashes, so I glance up seeing if I can examine its crystal pattern, but it melts too quickly. I kick at the snow gathering on the sidewalk. "They may not even be home for Christmas Eve dinner."

Kale stops, grabs my arms, and turns me to face him. "What?"

I feel tears prick my eyes, which is totally stupid, so I start walking again. "Yep. They may have," I make air quotes with my hands, "'school.'"

Kale falls in beside me. "I'm sorry, Poppie. I know you were planning a special night for your family. That sucks."

I wipe my eyes. "I don't really care. I'm not taking this class to make dinner for them anyway."

Kale grabs my arm and stops me again. "I can't believe I'm doing this because I know I'm going to regret it, but you're saying that your parents have a secret?"

"Yeah."

"Poppie." He gives me that look. "Your parents have a secret," he raises an eyebrow, "that you don't know."

Oh. Kale is so smart.

I feel a grin coming on. "And I love finding out secrets."

Kale nods and chuckles. "Yes, you do."

I inhale a deep breath of cold, snowy air, and suddenly feel invigorated. "Dude, you're so right. I'm good at finding out secrets, so I'm going to figure out theirs, and you're going to help me."

Kale shakes his head. "Pass."

He starts walking again, so I jog to catch up. "I know you're saying 'Pass,' but then I'll say 'Yes' and you'll say 'No,' and then I'll tell you a great story that will convince you to help me, so why don't we just skip past all that and you can agree to help me now?"

Kale laughs. "You know what I find weird? Investigating stuff doesn't sound like something your parents would do, but it is definitely right up your alley. As Miss Sweettarte would say, you can charm a secret out of a blazin' mad bull." He pauses in front of the revolving door going into Papa's Market. "I bet by the end of Papa's contest today you'll have charmed his secret out of him, too."

Oh no! The contest. I totally forgot about it.

I glance up at the sky. The snow is slowing and the sun is pushing through the clouds. It's an ideal day to be riding the slopes, or snowshoeing, or even shoveling the driveway. Anything would be better than going inside the market, losing a contest, and learning to cook a meal my parents aren't even going to eat.

I rub my forehead. "I'm not feeling so good."

Kale raises one dark eyebrow. "Why not?"

"I'm pretty sure I have malaria."

Kale snorts, not believing me for a second. "It's the dead of winter and all the mosquitoes are boogie boarding in Mexico. Come on. No more excuses."

Before I can argue, he pulls me into the revolving door next to him, and starts pushing. Our feet stumble over each other, and I can't help but laugh. We pass the opening into the market. I smell butter, cinnamon, and smoky wood. We propel ourselves around one more time before jumping out into the market.

Kale straightens his tie –it's covered in sparkly snow-flakes today- and then links his arm through mine. "Come on, in-fectious one, you owe me cookies from yesterday."

"Oh, you mean when you cheated?"

Kale acts shocked. "Cheated? I did no such thing."

We hurry to the back counter, stop a few feet short, unhook our arms, and take flying leaps onto our stools at the same time. It's a super loud double SCREEEE, and it's a moment I should remember forever so I decide to put Christmas Eve din-ner and my parents out of my mind. I'm just going to focus on en-joying whatever cookie Papa baked today.

"Papa?" I call out. "Anyone home?"

No answer. I search the front of the market, but don't see him. I'm about to call for him again when he scurries out of the kitchen. His brow is furrowed. His apron is crooked. And his bald head is sweating. He sets down two glasses of milk and a plate cradling two, oatmeal-raisin cookies. He doesn't say "Hi," doesn't give us time to say "Thanks," and forgets all about our thumb war before rushing back into the kitchen.

My mouth twists.

"That was odd," Kale comments.

I grab my glass to take a drink. It's warm. I gasp.

"Phwhat?" Kale mumbles through a mouthful of cookie.

I point to his glass. "Touch it."

His eyebrows shoot up. "It's not cold."

I bob my head. "Exactly! Papa has NEVER EVER brought us glasses that weren't ice cold."

Noises from the kitchen interrupt us.

BANG! CLATTER! POIIING!

Papa is tossing around pots, pans, and what looks like anything else he can find. He pauses for a few seconds, scratches his head, stares up at the ceiling, and then scratches his head again. He walks over to a shelf, lifts a bag of flour, peers under-neath it, and sets it down in a puff. He lifts up a big can on the next shelf, looks under it, and sets it back down with a clang.

I slap my hand on the counter. "He's lost something!"

Kale frowns at me. "That sounds like you, not Papa"

"What sounds like her?"

Ugh. That's a voice I'd love to forget.

Nick walks around to the kitchen side of the counter. He's dressed all in black again. Black jeans. Black sweater. But at least he's wearing the black cowboy boots instead of snowboarding boots. And he does look nice in that sweater.

Wait. What?

I shake my head. I'm not quite sure where that came from, but maybe I should be nice to him. It doesn't hurt to butter up the teacher's helper. Besides, maybe he was in a bad mood yesterday, or aliens abducted his body, and deep down he's really a nice guy.

I aim a huge, megawatt smile his way. "Well, look who's here! It's Papa's assistant!"

He looks like he's about to say something, but frowns when he sees my t-shirt, shakes his head, and walks back into the kitchen.

I turn to Kale and grin. "I'm pretty sure he really likes us."

Kale snorts, and points to my t-shirt. "I'm pretty sure he didn't like that."

"What's not to like about a cute pig?" I ask with a twinkle in my eye, already knowing the answer. It's possible I may have chosen today's shirt with Nick in mind. It has a cartoon pig lying on a beach blanket next to a slice of bacon. The caption above the pig reads:

I told you to put on sunscreen!

Clea shuffles up to the stool next to me.

I slap her on the back. "Hi, Pancake Queen."

"I don't know about that," she giggles as she sits down next to me and takes off her coat. She's wearing only one coat today, and her black hair is already back in a slick ponytail.

Li and Nacho walk up together.

"Yo, fellow chefs!" Li sings. She sits next to Kale and waves to Clea and me, making her snowboard earrings bounce.

Nacho sits on the stool next to Li. He's wearing another

red-and-blue soccer jersey with FCB on it. "I hope lunch today, it's good like yesterday! I'm starving."

I smile. This contest thing can't be so bad if I'm with these guys. Even if I do lose.

Then Tiffany arrives. She's wearing head-to-toe, pink-striped zebra, including the spaceship-sized beret on her head.

"Oh, hallo Nacho," she screeches as she takes the stool next to him, "if you're starving then why haven't you come to eat at my restaurant?"

Before Nacho can reply, Papa walks out of the kitchen. His eyebrows are drawn together and his eyes look like he's seen a ghost. And not a friendly one.

"Attention please," he bellows. "Welcome to your second day of *Yum Yum*. Nick will be covering the first part of the class." And without another word, he hurries back into the kitchen, picking up things and looking under them as he goes.

"He's definitely lost something," I whisper to Kale.

"I think you may be right," he murmurs.

"I think we need..."

Nick Clears his throat, interrupting me. "Shall I get started?"

I smile sweetly. "I'm so sorry. Please impress us with your Assistant-ness."

Nick rolls his eyes, and then probably to punish me, spends the next half-hour boring us to death with the names of all the different knives, utensils, and cooking equipment. As if we've never been in a kitchen before! Did he forget we were here yesterday? He does tell us about some clever substitutions, like using Greek yogurt instead of oil or sour cream, but I would eat fried crickets before I actually told him he was clever. But when he pulls out a bag of chocolate chips, I give him my full attention.

"Papa wanted to talk about mindful eating" Nick turns to face the kitchen. "Papa, we're ready when you are," he calls out before turning back to us. He passes out napkins, and gives us each two chocolate chips. "Please wait to eat these."

Two chocolate chips? Seems a little skimpy to me.

Papa returns, and I'm about to cheer until I see how unhappy he looks. His shoulders are slumped and deep lines wrinkle his forehead. Something is definitely wrong with him today, and I immediately wonder if The Suit visited him again.

"Great. Thanks, Nick." Papa motions to the chocolate chips in front of us. "Grab one chocolate chip and eat it as fast as you can."

I grab my teeny chip, chew it quickly, and swallow.

"Remember how that tasted," Papa advises. "Now I'm going to walk you through eating your other chocolate chip more mindfully. Eat only half of it, and as you slowly chew that half, really take the time to savor it. Imagine this is the last piece of chocolate on Earth, and you get to enjoy it. Focus on the sweet flavor and the creamy texture. When you swallow, think about what memory it brings to your mind?"

Laughing with Kale when we ate Papa's chocolaty Triple-Chocolate Cookies yesterday.

"Now eat the other half," Papa continues. "Just as slowly and mindfully. How does it make you feel?"

Happy. Really warm and happy.

Papa continues. "Now which chocolate chip did you enjoy? The first one you ate quickly and not mindfully? Or the second one where you really savored every bite and every wonderful flavor?"

I raise my hand. "Definitely the second one."

Li nods. "I agree. It was weird because I know the two chocolate chips were exactly the same, but I think the mindful one tasted much better!"

I nod in agreement. "It was almost like I ate two totally different chocolate chips. The first one was good, but the second one was way better."

"Why do you think that is?" Papa asks.

I think for a second. "Eating slower made the flavors really explode in my mouth. And it seemed like I was eating way more chocolate than that itty-bitty chocolate chip."

Papa nods. "I believe eating mindfully is one of the greatest secrets to healthy eating. When we eat food in front of the TV or rushing out the door, we don't really focus on what we're eating and it doesn't taste as good. But when we eat mindfully and savor our food, we feel more satisfied and eat less."

Interesting. I'm about to suggest we test his theory with more chocolate chips, but Papa is ready to move on.

He hands us each a packet. "Today we're making lunch. I made a big pot of my favorite vegetable soup to go with sandwiches and salads that you will all make. Same groups grab the same dry and cold ingredients, and then everyone meet at the workstation."

My brave Team Refrigerator has no problem with the door this time because I put myself in charge of holding it open. As I set my last load of ingredients on the workstation, Kale sidles up next to me.

"Papa assigned us to work together today" he says with a grin.

I salute him. "Chef Burn reporting for duty."

Kale tilts his head. "Although Chef Burn does have a nice ring to it, I'm afraid your amazing blackening powers will not be needed today. There's nothing to burn. Only sandwiches to assemble."

I whoop and fist punch the air. "I can totally make a sammie!"

Kale hands me a package of mozzarella. "Then you can cut the cheese," he says with a sly grin.

I raise my eyebrows. "I don't think that's a good idea in this enclosed space."

Nick happens to stroll by right at that moment. "What's not a good idea?"

"Cutting the cheese," I giggle.

Nick gives me a funny look before enlightenment dawns on his face. I swear I see a hint of a grin before he shakes his head and walks away.

"You're a goof," Kale laughs.

I punch him in the arm. "Right back at ya, dude." I grab the mozzarella. "I don't think this cheese wants to be sliced."

"Why?"

I grin. "Because it has grater plans!"

Kale and I manage to amuse ourselves with cheesy jokes while we assemble the sandwiches. We bring our *Mozzie Tom Sammies* up to the checkerboard counter, and set them next to a big pot of *Papa's Favorite Vegetable Soup*, a plate of *Tuna, Berries & Greens* and a bowl of *Cornie Quinoa*.

Everything looks so delicious that my stomach grumbles. Loudly.

Kale punches me.

I shrug. "I can't help it." I turn to Papa. "When do we get to dig in?"

He stares at me for a moment, as if confused by my question, but then nods and waves his hand. "Yes, go ahead. I... um. I'll be back in a moment."

I'm really wondering what's up with him today, but my stomach wins over my brain. I want to overload my plate, but I remember what Papa said about eating slower making us feel fuller, so I take a little of everything. I can always go back for seconds if he's totally wrong, and I'm still hungry.

Papa doesn't reappear, so Nick reviews our creations.

"Let's start with *Papa's Favorite Vegetable Soup*," he says. "I've heard from a few of you that you love when he makes this soup, especially on a cold day. But did you know that it's healthy? The vegetables and potatoes provide vitamins, minerals, and fiber, and the beans give it protein."

"Now to the *Mozzie Tom Sammies*," he continues. "A quick but healthy lunch option when you're short on time. Using whole wheat bread assures you have fiber to keep you satisfied longer, and olive oil is full of healthy fats. You can even do an open face sandwich with one slice of bread if you want to save a few calories." He looks at Kale and I. "Great job on the sammies. The olive oil and balsamic ratio is perfect."

I almost fall off my stool. A compliment from Red? And he

laughed at our cutting-the-cheese joke. What is happening? Is the world ending, and I don't know it?

Nick continues his review. "Next, we have the *Tuna, Berries & Greens*. This is a great post-workout lunch because tuna gives a huge punch of protein while the berries, walnuts, and greens give us antioxidants to combat the stresses of exercise." He smiles at Nacho and Li. "Great job, you two."

He moves on. "And then we have the *Cornie Quinoa*. It takes a little extra prep time, but quinoa is a fantastic grain because it has complete proteins, which is great for vegetarians, and even for non-vegetarians. It's high in fiber and protein, and adding in the beans and vegetables gives it even more fiber which helps us feel fuller longer. Good job on the dressing, Clea and Tiffany."

I guess he had to include Tiffany, but I'm pretty sure she did nothing but text away on her phone while Clea was cooking. And how does he know all about ants and oxidants, or whatever he said? He must take being Papa's assistant very serious. Or it's just the end of the world thing.

I finish what's on my plate and debate going back for seconds of quinoa, but decide I'm actually full and feel quite satisfied. Papa was right. Mindful eating does work.

We finish cleaning (Tiffany threw a few napkins away), and are heading back to the counter when Papa joins us again.

"Good job today." Papa tries to smile, but it doesn't really reach his eyes. "We're finishing up early today, but before you leave, I want to review something. What does a good chef include when planning a healthy meal?"

"Beef?" Li offers.

Papa extends his pointer finger. "Right. A Protein. It can be beef, chicken, or fish, but it can also be beans, legumes, quinoa, nuts, or dairy." He holds up a second finger. "What else do we need?"

"Fruit," Li says.

"Vegetable," Kale says at the same time.

Papa nods and extends two more fingers.

"Starchy," Nacho says hesitantly.

Papa raises another finger. "A starch. Yes, good. And let's call the starch a Whole Grain. So, we need Protein, Fruit, Vegetable, and Whole Grain to create a healthy meal."

"You forgot one," I remark with a mischievous smile.

Papa raises one bushy, white eyebrow. "I did?"

I nod, my braids flying. "The most important one. Cookies!"

Everyone laughs. Papa even cracks a real smile.

"Of course. Cookies. There's always room for dessert." He reaches under the counter and sets one white, bakery bag in front of each of us. "This is your homework for tomorrow. It's a contest of sorts, so wait to open them until after I leave. No cooking is involved, but you do have to plan." He smiles at me before continuing. "Two things I want you all to remember for this homework. The best meals are a little healthy and a little treat, a smidge of tweaking, and a lot of love. *And* a good chef is only as good as those helping him or her. Good luck, everyone. See you tomorrow."

We only have to plan? No cooking? And this is the contest? I almost jump on the counter and do a happy dance right there. This is great! I'm awesome at planning!

Papa tells us goodbye and bustles off to the front of the market.

Nick starts to follow him, but Tiffany latches onto his arm, whispering something in his ear. He smiles and nods, and as they walk past me I hear her whisper, "Now, I can finally make them. And you can help me, Nick Sweettarte."

I gag. I don't even want to know what they're talking about.

"Anybody up for some hot chocolate?" Li offers. "We can check out what's in our homework bags."

Nacho nods. "More chocolate is good to me."

"I second that," Kale agrees.

"Clea and Poppie, you have time to hang with us?" Li asks.

I nod. "Homework is always more fun with friends."

Clea looks a little hesitant, but nods in agreement.

Everyone grabs their bags, and heads towards the fireplace.

I grab Kale's arm. "Hold up a second."

He looks at me with confusion. "What's wrong?"

I wait until the others are out of earshot. "Something is going on with Papa today, and it's really bugging me. I think he may need our help."

Kale snorts. "Our help? Or your prying?"

I act shocked. "What? Me? I have absolutely no idea what you are talking about." I point to the grocery where Papa is frantically looking under every item on every shelf. He suddenly looks wide-eyed right at us.

"That's a scary look," Kale whispers.

Papa rushes towards us, skirts around the counter and ducks to the ground.

I peek over the counter. "Hey, Papa, you okay?"

Papa doesn't look up from searching the shelves. "Sure. Just busy."

"You look like you're tearing apart your market. And that's what I do when I lose something. Is something lost?" Never hurts to ask.

Papa looks up at us, his eyes a little wild. "I know I put it there. I know for sure that I did." He exhales a long sigh. "But now it's gone."

Kale leans over the counter and peers down at Papa. "What's gone?"

Papa's forehead is so furrowed with wrinkles that it reminds me of a walnut. His sits back on the floor, and shakes his head. "I don't know if I should tell you."

"We could help you look," I offer. "I'm really amazing at searching because I lose things all the time."

Kale nods. "It's true. No one loses things more than Poppie."

"Please let us help you," I beg. "With three of us looking, we're bound to find whatever it is you lost."

Kale chuckles. "Better to just say yes, Papa, because you know she won't stop until you let her help."

Papa laughs. A real laugh. "Okay, okay." He gestures to the back of the kitchen. "But let's go back to my office. If you're going to help me look, first I need to tell you my secret."

His secret?

All I want for Christmas is... this!

CHAPTER 11

Papa Tells Us His Secret

I'm surprised at the state of Papa's office. It reminds me of my bedroom- chaotic, messy, and not at all organized. Piles of starched napkins and plastic-wrapped aprons clutter his desk. Stacked, empty boxes teeter in every corner and loose papers litter the floor, the chairs, and the walls.

Papa picks up a folder burping receipts off a chair and dumps it on the floor. "Please, sit down." He walks around the desk, chucks an empty cardboard box off his chair, and plops down. "I feel like I've searched everywhere, but I still can't find it."

"What is *it*?" I ask, sitting down. Kale leans on the armrest.

Before Papa can answer, I hear an arrogant voice behind us.

"I thought I'd find you here,"

I twist around and see The Suit standing in the doorway.

Papa leans back in his chair, and frowns. "I'm sorry, but I'm in a meeting right now."

The Suit waves his bony hand. "That's ok. This will only take a moment." He sneers down his long nose at Kale and me, and then smooths his dark hair in that odd angle across his eyes. "I'm sure this meeting is not important as my business."

Papa stands up, walks around the desk, and tries to usher

The Suit out the door. "It is important, so I am busy right now."

"Too busy to save your store?" The Suit scoffs.

What?

Papa glances at us. "Excuse me for a moment." He glares at The Suit. "Please follow me," he orders, and leads him out the door.

I stare wide-eyed at Kale. I'm about to freak out about why The Suit said Papa needs to save his store when I hear Papa's angry voice.

"Why have you returned? I told you I'm not interested in your client's offer, and I never will be."

"I highly recommend you reconsider his offer," The Suit sniffs, "because if you don't, he will see to it that your market has a quick demise."

Demise? As in death? What the heck?

"Are you threatening me?" Papa growls.

The Suit Clears his throat. "I will give you until tomorrow to reconsider. Good day to you."

Kale and I stare at each other in shock. Is this Papa's secret? Is he going to lose his market? He loves his market. We love his market. Butte wouldn't be the same without it.

Papa walks back in looking as angry as a bull elk protecting his herd. "I'm assuming you heard all that."

It's not a question, but we both nod.

He sighs, and plops back into his chair. "I'd appreciate it if you didn't tell anyone what you heard. This is nothing to be worried about. Okay?"

"But Papa, why did he say…" I start to ask, but Papa interrupts me.

"Poppie, please." He holds up his hands. "This is my business and not yours, okay?"

I've never seen him this serious, so I zip it and nod.

He rubs his forehead. "So, now back to my real problem. Poppie, you were right. I've lost something. Something very important to me."

I give him my most serious look. "Don't worry, we'll help

you find it."

I hate seeing him so upset. And if this "real" problem isn't about the fact that someone is trying to shut down his market, it must be really bad.

Papa smiles. "I know you will." He stands up. "I've lost the box of chocolate that I used to make *Papa's Triple-Chocolate Cookies* cookies yesterday."

"Even though it wasn't my birthday!" I add.

"Or that holiday called Valentine's Day," Kale smirks.

Papa nods. "Yes. Usually, I can only get that certain chocolate in February, but I found a new supplier who delivered a box a few days ago, and now that chocolate is gone." He throws his arms into the air. "Gone! Just gone."

"Can you just order another box?" Kale asks.

"I did. But it won't be here for a week, and I need that chocolate tomorrow." Papa shakes his head. "I just don't know what happened to it. One minute it was here and the next it was gone. Poof. Disappeared."

I suddenly remember Nick's strange behavior yesterday. "Or someone took it."

Papa tilts his head. "Why would someone take it?"

I'm so excited that I jump up from the chair. "I bet Nick took it. Yesterday I saw him sneak out of the kitchen hiding something in his jacket." I slam my hands on his desk. "I bet it was your box of chocolate!"

Papa doesn't look surprised anymore. "Was this right before I started class?"

"Yes!"

He shakes his head. "That was just a bag of socks."

My mouth drops open. "What?"

Kale chuckles. "Socks?"

Papa nods. "Yes, I had just given them to him. He's collecting warm clothing to send to the troops."

"For the troops?" I ask, totally confused. Why would Nick be doing something nice like that? I don't believe it. I raise one eyebrow. "If it was just a bag of socks, then why was he trying to hide it?"

Papa shrugs. "I have an idea, but that's not for me to say. If you get to know him a bit more, maybe you'll find out, too." He stands. "If you would like to help me search for the chocolate, I'd be very grateful." He holds his hands about a foot apart. "It's in a box about the size of a shoebox. It's dark brown, with white cursive on the side. I'll search the grocery again if you two can really scour the kitchen."

Kale and I follow Papa out of the office. He returns to the front of the market while Kale and I let the others know we can't join them. I tell them we're helping Papa and luckily they don't ask why.

Kale and I search every inch of the kitchen. We even crawl around on our hands and knees to look under shelves. After searching for almost thirty minutes, we meet Papa back in his office.

"Well?" he asks.

I plunk down into the chair, and shake my head. "No luck."

Kale frowns. "I'm sorry, Papa"

Papa slumps into his chair. "I think it's time I just accept that it's gone." He sighs. "This definitely throws a kink in my Christmas Eve."

I sit up straighter. "Christmas Eve? Why?"

"It's another secret." He shrugs. "But I guess it doesn't really matter anymore because now I have to cancel."

"Then you can tell us."

Kale shakes his head. "Poppie."

Papa waves him off. "No worries, Kale. It doesn't matter anymore since I can't do it anyway." He gives us a dimpled half-smile. "I was going to surprise Miss Sweettarte with her favorite dessert during our Christmas Eve dinner."

I'm starting to understand. "*Papa's Triple-Chocolate Cookies.*"

Papa nods. "And then I was going to give her a ring, and…"

I can't help it. I interrupt him. "A ring?!"

Papa manages a weak smile. "Yes. I was going to ask her to

marry me."

"Marry you?!" I shout.

Papa Shortdough wants to marry Miss Sweettarte? I love Papa Shortdough! I love Miss Sweettarte! I can't think of two nicer people who should be together and live happily ever after!

I jump out of my chair and leap up and down, my braids bouncing like popcorn in a skillet. "This is so exciting!"

Papa shakes his head and looks even more miserable than before. "No, it's not."

I stop jumping. "Why?"

"Because I'm not going to ask her."

I tilt my head. "Why not? Because you're a grandpa?"

Kale thumps me in the arm. "No! Because he doesn't have the chocolate and he can't make the *Triple-Chocolate Cookies*!"

Kale's so smart.

I wave my hands. "That doesn't matter. You're Papa Shortdough, Chef Extraordinaire! You can just create a new dessert! Then it can always remind you lovebirds of the night you got engaged, and you can call it, When-I-asked-You-to-Marry-Me-and-You-Said-Yes Dessert!"

Kale snorts. "Cause that's easy to say."

Papa shakes his head. "You don't understand."

"But I do! I know Miss Sweettarte likes you so much that she'll say yes even if you don't make *Papa's Triple-Chocolate Cookies*!" I grab one of the napkins off the desk and put it on my head like a veil. I titter like Miss Sweettarte and try to copy her southern drawl. "Why, yes, Papa Shortdough, I'd be tickled pink to marry you!" I wiggle the fingers on my left hand and whisper. "Now you put the sparkly ring on my finger."

Papa looks like he's about to puke. I didn't think my impression of Miss Sweettarte was that bad.

"I can't," he says miserably.

"You can't put a ring on a finger?" Sometimes I wonder how adults survive in this world.

Papa takes a very long and very deep breath. "I can't, because I don't have the ring. I put it into the box of chocolate to keep it safe."

I fall into the chair. "And that box is missing."

He nods. "Yep. The very same one."

Oh, Jingle Bells.

CHAPTER 12

I Know Who Stole The Box

I frown. "The ring you were going to give Miss Sweettarte is in the missing box of chocolate?"

Papa Shortdough taps his nose.

This is a pickle. I absolutely adore Papa Shortdough. He's the nicest man in this town and he deserves to live happily ever after with Miss Sweettarte. There has to be a way I can help.

"I've never been married." I jerk my thumb toward Kale. "Unless you count that time my dog married Kale and me when we were ten. But I don't think you need a ring to be happily married. My dad didn't have a ring when he asked my mom to marry him, and they've been married twenty years!"

I think I see a tiny light of hope flicker in Papa's eyes. He strokes his chin. He stands up and paces. Back and forth. Back and forth. Then WHAM! He pounds his fist on the desk. "Poppie, you're right!"

I grin. "So, you're going to ask her?"

He beams at me and nods, happy crinkles appearing at the corners of his eyes.

I rub my hands together. "Then it's time to start planning..."

He holds up his hands. "Wait a minute, Poppie. Thanks

for helping me, but I would like to take it from here." He grabs our bakery bags off his desk and hands them over. "And you two need to skedaddle. You have homework."

I take my bag. "You sure you don't need any help?" I grin. "You know I'm excellent at making plans"

Papa chuckles. "Yes, you are. Thank you for the offer, but this is something I want to do myself. But, will you both please promise to keep this a secret?"

Kale and I pinky-promise, and leave Papa in his office. We walk out of the kitchen and find Li, Nacho, and Clea sitting at the checkerboard counter.

"Yo!" Li calls out. She motions to the white bakery bag sitting in front of her. "Have you opened your bags yet?"

I shake my head.

"Check this out." She pulls a piece of paper out of her bag and sets it on the counter. It's a photograph of a head of lettuce.

I laugh. "That's what's in our bags? A picture of lettuce?"

Li shakes her head. "Nope. That's what's in my bag." She motions to Nacho and Clea. "These guys have something different."

Nacho pulls out a photo of a carrot, and Clea pulls out a photo of an apple.

"We were wondering what's in your bags," Li asks.

Kale opens his bag and pulls out the paper. "Mine is bread."

I peek into my bag and burst out laughing. I pull the paper out for everyone to see.

"It's a rubber chicken." Kale snorts. "Classic Papa."

Clea organizes the photos on the counter. "Papa Shortdough said we had to do a little planning. We have a fruit, two vegetables, bread, and a chicken." She taps each one. "Maybe...," she stops and shakes her head.

I raise my eyebrows. "Maybe what?"

Her cheeks flush. "I'm not sure. It's just a guess."

Li sits down next to Clea and puts her arm around her. "Tell us, girlfriend! A guess is better than nothing, which is what

I have."

Clea doesn't look up but quickly says, "I think Papa Short-dough wants us to plan a healthy meal using these foods."

Li nods thoughtfully. "Yeah. I think you're right! Papa Shortdough said a good chef is only as good as those who help him or her. I think we all have to work together to plan a dinner."

Clea frowns. "Except we're missing Tiffany and whatever her food is."

"We could text her," Kale says.

I almost punch him.

Li shakes her head. "We can't. She's in flight to Aspen with her parents." She winks at Nacho. "She even invited our fútbol star here to go along on their private jet, and he politely refused."

Nacho shrugs. "I think she asked Nick to go, too."

I'm suddenly grinning ear-to-ear. Both Tiffany and Nick are gone? I envision our class tomorrow without them where all of us are dancing with unicorns and sliding down rainbows.

Until Nacho shatters my dream.

"We can ask her tomorrow," he says. "She say she will be back tonight for dinner at restaurant."

The rainbow fades and the unicorns fly away.

Kale drums his fingers on the counter. "But we can't plan a meal without knowing what her photo is."

"I heard her tell Nick something about chocolate cookies," Li offers. "So maybe it's chocolate?"

Chocolate?

Something gnaws at the back of my brain. Something about chocolate? When Tiffany walked out with Nick today weren't they talking about chocolate?

OH! MY! GOSH!

I grab Kale's arm. "Tiffany took the box!"

Kale's eyes widen.

Oops. My bad. I'm not supposed to say anything. I pinky-promised.

I chuckle. "Right. What I meant was that Tiffany probably has a picture of a box of chocolate in her bag." I start shuffling the food photos and pretend to be very interested in them. "So, anyone know a good recipe for rubber chicken?"

Li saves me without even knowing it. "I bet we could find one on the Internet!"

While everyone searches for recipes on their phones, all I can think about is Tiffany. I just know she stole Papa's box of chocolate! She must be using it to make cookies like she told Nick. But how did she take it? And where is it now?

After what feels like an entire school year has passed, we finally finish the menu.

"I can print the recipes and bring them in tomorrow," Clea volunteers.

"Great," I say, probably too loudly. I grab Kale's arm and tug him toward the door. "Well, we better get going. We promised my parents we'd... um... clean the carpet today."

Kale's eyebrows pop up. "We did?"

"Yes!" I pinch his arm.

"OW!"

I pull Kale through the market, push him into the revolving door, and follow him outside.

He looks confused. "Are we really cleaning your carpet?"

I shake my head. "No. We're going over to C'est La Ski to demand that Tiffany gives back Papa's box of chocolate!"

I wait for an SUV to pass and then dart across the street. I'm marching with a purpose and a plan towards the restaurant when Kale catches up with me.

"But Tiffany's not there," he reminds me.

Oh. Dang.

Rudolph with your nose so bright, we need a new plan tonight.

CHAPTER 13

Mister Protein and Miss Icy

I'm sitting on a bench in the ladies locker room at The Rock, holding three-inch, red heels, and wishing I had grabbed the sensible, black flats from Kale's mom's closet.

I glance at my watch. It's already 3:45 PM. We only have an hour before Berg picks us up so I suck it up, slip on the shoes, and check myself out in the mirror.

Kale and I borrowed clothes from his parents' closet, and are trying to look like producers from the very popular *Foodie Show* on You Tube. I've hidden my long braids under a white beret, wrapped myself in a polar-bear-worthy, white sweater dress, and left on my rainbow-colored knee socks. I smeared blue shadow over my eyelids, all the way up to my eyebrows, and used it to fill in my lips. I think I look like a hip snow fairy with wicked red heels.

I take my first wobbly step, and immediately regret my decision. My ankles buck and twist like a bronco at the rodeo and throw me to the floor.

I giggle. That was fun. But I can't wear these if I expect to actually walk anywhere. I take them off, and head out of the locker room to meet Kale.

He busts out laughing the second he sees me. "The rainbow socks," he laughs. "And that blue all over your eyes and lips." He points to his white suit and the red ski hat on his head. "I'm pretty boring compared to you."

I hold up the blue shadow. "Not for long. And it matches that lovely blue, ruffled tie you're wearing."

Kale shakes his head.

I nod.

He shakes his head again.

I nod.

He rolls his eyes. "Fine. But not too much. I don't know how you keep talking me into these things," he grumbles.

"Dude, it's for Papa."

He sighs. "I know. And that's the only reason I'm letting you do this."

A few people give us funny looks as I smear blue all over his lips and eyelids.

He purses his mouth like a model, and asks in a deep voice. "How do I look?"

"Fabulous!" I laugh. "The blue really pops against your beautiful, dark skin. Like an icy masterpiece!"

He rolls his eyes again, but blushes just a little. "Oh, huge pass." He holds out his arm. "Shall we?"

I link my arm in his. "Yes, Mister Protein, let us away to the restaurant."

Kale raises his eyebrows. "Protein?"

"It is *The Foodie Show*."

We stroll arm in arm out of the resort and onto the side-walk. We could get to C'est La Ski from inside the resort, but we want to make a grand entrance at the front door. I'm pretty sure the blue eyeshadow will help us with that.

The sun has already slipped behind the mountain. And even though the melted snow on the sidewalk is starting to freeze again, my socks are soon soaked through and my feet are frozen by the time we reach the restaurant. It's officially not open for dinner yet, but luckily the door is unlocked.

"Wait a second," I tell Kale when he reaches to open the door. "I have to put my shoes back on." I lean on his arm and slip on the heels, hoping I can magically walk in them now.

Kale opens the door and bows. "Ladies first."

"Why thank you, kind sir." I sashay past him, immediately catch my heel on the rug, and stumble right into the receptionist desk. My dress is so tight that I'm stuck lying at an angle against the desk, like a frozen fluffy white statue in rainbow socks.

Kale rushes in to help me at the same time a waiter in a black tuxedo rushes over. He opens his mouth to speak but nothing comes out. I'm pretty sure it's the blue eyeshadow.

Kale greets the waiter. "Aye, Matey, today's your lucky day, my good lad!"

My eyes pop open. Why is he talking like an Irish pirate? I give him a wide-eyed look, and mouth "no pirate."

Kale laughs. "Just kidding around with some show biz fun! Allow us to introduce ourselves. This is Miss Icy and I am Mister Protein."

I'm about to say hello when I realize I'm slowly sliding down the front of the receptionist desk. In fact, I'm going to be doing push-ups on the floor very soon if Kale doesn't help me.

"Mister Protein, would you be so kind as to help me up?" I yelp as calmly as I can.

Kale jumps forward, grabs me under my shoulders and pulls me up.

I straighten my dress and frown at the waiter. "We're here to scout your restaurant for *The Foodie Show*, *if* you will ever let us in?"

The mention of the world famous, cooking show seems to finally jolt the waiter out of his shock. "I'm so sorry." He blinks a few times. "Mademoiselle. Monsieur. Please, come in."

I tentatively take a step, wobble way too much, and promptly lurch into the waiter. We stagger across the restaurant, crash into a table, and drag the tablecloth with us as we fall to the marble floor, silverware clattering all around us.

Kale rushes over, grabs my arm and yanks me up, holding me tight to his side.

I tuck my braids back into my beret. "Mr. Waiter Guy, we're wasting time with all these games," I huff.

The waiter is lying face down. He rolls over and stares wide-eyed at the ceiling. You'd think he'd just been hit by a truck. Or a robust girl. I do know how to make an entrance.

I put my hands on my hips. "Now, will you kindly show us your pantry, or do you want to keep playing?"

"Of course, Mademoiselle," he says crisply as he slowly stands up. He straightens his jacket. "I would be happy to show you...," he pauses and looks at me with raised eyebrows. "The pantry? Would you not like to see the kitchen first?"

I scream inside. We're wasting time! We need to search for the box of chocolate before Tiffany and her parents get back from Aspen, and I know the pantry has to be the best place to look.

I wave my hand to dismiss his question. "Of course, we shall see the kitchen, but first we must inspect the pantry."

The waiter takes a long look at me before he answers. "I do not recall a Miss Icy or a Mister Protein on the show. And I believe the show would call ahead to arrange this visit." He narrows his eyes. "And I believe you are *not* with *The Foodie Show*."

Oh, you're a mean one, Mr. Grinch.

CHAPTER 14

We Find More Than Powdered Sugar

My plan won't work if this waiter doesn't believe us. I debate grabbing Kale and hightailing it out of there, but I know we can't back out now. We have to help Papa.

I let out an exaggerated sigh, roll my eyes and turn to Kale. "Why must I deal with amateurs?"

Kale pats my hand. "Now, now Miss Icy. I'm certain this young man will be very accommodating." He tsks. "I know he would hate for Mr. and Mrs. Bouffe to find out their restaurant wasn't on our show because of him."

The waiter's eyes widen ever so slightly. I can see he's mulling it over, weighing his options. Should I believe these crazy people, or risk being fired? He must decide not to mess with the Bouffe's wrath because he frowns and says, "I apologize. Please follow me to the pantry."

I hold on to Kale's arm for balance, and we follow the waiter through a swinging door and smack dab into the middle of the bustling kitchen. Six people are frantically prepping for the dinner rush. Knives whoosh through vegetables. Whisks clink against metal bowls. Water boils in huge pots on the stove. I hope we can sneak past, but the waiter has a different idea. He stops right in the middle of the kitchen.

"May I present Mister Protein and Miss Icy from *The Foodie Show*," he announces so formally that he must think we are the Duke and Duchess of Blue Eyeshadow Land.

The kitchen comes to a standstill, and all eyes settle on us.

I lift my chin higher. Kale waves like he's in a parade.

"Hello, all! Nice to be here," Kale says. He winks at a short, squat man in a towering chef's hat. "Can't wait to see what's for dinner."

The man narrows his eyes. He's wearing the tallest hat so does that mean he's the head chef or just the shortest? Either way he doesn't look happy that we're interrupting prep time.

"Time to move along." I whisper to Kale out of the corner of my mouth.

Kale grins broadly. "Please return to your efforts." He motions to the waiter. "Lead on, kind sir."

Kale grabs my arm again to help me walk, and we follow the waiter across the kitchen and down a short hallway. I'm looking over my shoulder to see if we're being followed when Kale suddenly pulls me to a stop. I whip my head around to find myself inches from the waiter's face.

His eyebrows pop up.

I grin. "Well, hello there!"

His eyes widen, but he doesn't step back. Impressive.

He opens a door beside him and motions inside. "Our pantry."

It's a massive walk-in that's half the size of my dining room with four shelves full of boxes, bags and cans. That's a lot of food to look through. We're going to need time to search. Alone.

I try to dismiss the waiter by waving my hand. We're still standing almost nose-to-nose. "Thank you. We'll take it from here."

"I shall remain to answer any questions, Mademoiselle."

I frown. We can't steal back the box of chocolate if he's standing here watching our every move.

I suddenly have an idea. I close my eyes. "Ohm," I chant. "Ohm." I start swaying like I've seen my mom do when she meditates sometimes. "Ohmmmm. Ohmmmm. UGH!" I open my eyes. My chanting must have frightened the waiter because he's moved a few steps away from me.

I point my finger at him. "I can't work with you here. I cannot feel the ingredients. You're disturbing my aura." I point to the hallway. "Please go!"

I can feel Kale shaking with laughter, but he swallows it. "Sorry, but you do *not* want to know what happens if her aura is disturbed. You better go, and we'll let you know when we're finished here."

The waiter opens his mouth to speak. I shake my head.

He raises his eyebrows. I hold up my hand.

He narrows his eyes. I shove my hands on my hips, scrunch every muscle in my face, and bare my teeth like I've seen Lucy do when other dogs threaten her.

I must make an impression because the waiter's eyes widen in fear before he scurries down the hallway and around the corner.

Kale starts laughing so hard he can't talk.

I giggle. "Good, huh?"

He nods. "I just can't believe he's buying it," he whispers. "I thought he was gonna kick us out the minute you crashed into the table."

I chuckle. "Me, too. Glad he was there to break my fall." I let go of Kale, hold onto the doorframe, and take a wobbly step into the pantry. "You look on that side. Papa's box of chocolate has got to be in here somewhere!"

I search the bottom shelf. Canned tomatoes. Boxes of pasta. Bags of garlic. No chocolate. I search the next shelf. Spices. Spices. More spices. The third shelf is full of jars. Anchovies. Roasted peppers. And what looks like whole squid. Yuck!

I'm tall, but not tall enough to see what's up on the top shelf. I look around. No stools or ladders. I hold onto a middle shelf for support, balance on my spiky heels, and reach up with my hand to feel around.

Of course, this doesn't work.

As I fall, my hand tries to grab onto a bag of something, knocking it off the shelf and onto the floor, exploding white powder all over the pantry.

I lick my lips. Powdered sugar.

"You okay?" Kale asks.

"Yeah." I'm just about to ask if he thinks anyone heard me crash, when the chef appears at the door.

He throws up his hands. "What is zis?!"

I don't answer. *Zis* is not part of my plan.

The waiter appears. His mouth rounds into a big O before he covers it with both hands. "I told you they were not professionals!"

The chef taps his foot and glares at me.

I chortle. "This is... um... well... you see.... I forgot my perfume and wanted to smell a bit sweeter." I give them what I think is a megawatt smile.

"Hallo!"

I stiffen at the familiar shrill voice that is way too close. Kale's eyes grow wide.

"Hallo?" Tiffany calls out again. "Chef Pierre?"

Time for us to skedaddle. And fast!

Kale grabs the chef's hand and pumps it. "Congratulations! You're in the top five, Matey." He grabs my arm and yanks me out the door.

Kale supports me as we race around the corner. We've just reached the kitchen when we hear Tiffany ask, "Who was that?"

I stop Kale. "Wait." I reach down, unlatch my heels, and yank them off. My big thighs can run much faster without these spiky death traps. "Let's get out of here!" I squeal.

Kale races out the swinging door, and I follow close behind. We run through the dining room and out the restaurant's side door that leads into the resort. The ski lifts have just closed for the night so a sea of colorful jackets, snowboards, and skis immediately engulfs us. I almost cheer. The crowd will hide us!

I glance back at the door leading into the restaurant, only to see the chef and waiter tumble out, scan the crowd, and then – YIKES! - point in our direction!

I yank the red hat off Kale's head. "Duck down! And run!" I scrunch down as short as I can, and dash in and out of the crowd with Kale on my heels. When we reach the locker rooms, I risk a peek behind us. I don't see the chef or waiter. "Change!" I hiss to Kale. He nods and races into the men's locker room.

I slam my shoulder into the door and dart inside the ladies locker room. I jerk open the locker, grab my backpack, and dash into a stall. I quickly change back into my jeans and sweater, shake the remaining sugar out of Kale's mom's clothes, and stuff it all into my backpack.

I crack open the stall door and glance around. The locker room is crowded with gals comparing their runs. No chef. No waiter. No Tiffany.

I exit the stall and find an open sink. I get a couple odd looks as I scrub the blue off my eyes and lips, but no one says anything. When I think every trace of Miss Icy is gone, I peek out of the locker room door and see Kale sitting on a bench, back in his jeans and tie.

I walk out, and sit down beside him. I giggle. "Well, that was fun."

He chuckles. "Surprisingly, yes."

"But useless." I sigh.

Kale grins. "I wouldn't say useless." He pulls a piece of paper out of his pocket. "I did find this."

My heartbeat quickens. I look at him with wide eyes. "Where did you get that?"

"I saw it laying on the counter in the kitchen while you were taking off your shoes." He grins even wider. "So, I grabbed it."

I can't believe it. Rule-following Kale stole something.

And it's a recipe for *Papa's Triple-Chocolate Cookies*.

I think it's going to be a very, merry Christmas.

CHAPTER 15

I Have a Revelation

W e race into Papa's Market and find him adding logs to his massive fireplace.

"Papa!" I yell as we screech to a stop behind him.

I must sound panicked because he turns around with concern in his eyes. "Poppie. Kale. What's wrong?"

"We need to talk to you in private. It's important!"

He motions around him at the empty couches. "I think this is pretty private."

I glance around. I didn't even notice that the market is dark and totally deserted. That's odd. At four o'clock it's usually jam-packed with people who have just come off the slopes.

"Where is everyone?" Kale asks.

Papa sighs. "Hopefully, somewhere warm."

I can't wait any longer. The news bursts out of me. "Tiffany stole your chocolate!"

Papa frowns. "What?"

"She stole it to make *Papa's Triple-Chocolate Cookies!*"

"Are you sure?"

"Positive!"

Papa shakes his head. "Wait a minute. A couple hours ago you thought Nick stole my chocolate."

"I know. I was wrong." I pause for a minute. "Unless he helped her steal it and then she took it to C'est La Ski." I hand him the recipe.

He looks at it, and then back at me. "Where did you get this?"

I look at Kale. He shakes his head slightly. I've known him long enough that I understand what he means. Just tell the edited version. The details are likely to get us into trouble.

"I…um…I think the less you know the better." I point to the recipe. "But that recipe was in the kitchen at C'est La Ski!"

Papa chortles. "And this is why you think they have my chocolate?"

He's laughing?! I'm stunned. "Yeah! Why else would they have your secret cookie recipe that no one else in the world has?"

Papa sits down on the couch. "Tiffany's parents have been trying to copy my triple-chocolate cookies for years." He shows us the recipe. "Look at all those question marks and eraser smudges. This is not my recipe. This is a copycat they're trying to create." He chuckles. "And they're not even close."

"But she took your chocolate!" I argue.

"You saw her with it?"

I bite my fingernail. "Well…no."

He nods as if that's the end of it. But I'm not ready to give up.

"I just know she has it!" I start pacing. "After class today, Tiffany told Nick that she had the chocolate so she could finally make the cookies! And Li heard her, too!" I stop in front of Papa.. "She had to be talking about your cookies! Now all you have to do is go to C'est La Ski, demand they give you back your box of chocolate, get your ring," I throw my arms out to the side, "and ta da, you can propose to Miss Sweettarte!" I grin at my sweet plan that will fix everything.

Papa doesn't return my smile. "Did you see my box of chocolate in C'est La Ski?"

My smile slides into a frown. "No," I mumble.

"I know you're trying to help, but I won't accuse someone of stealing without proof."

I sit down next to him and point to the recipe. "But this is proof!"

Papa shakes his head. "No. This is just an attempt to copy a recipe. It's not proof Tiffany took my chocolate."

I narrow my eyes. "Okay, then. New plan. I'll find you proof." I stand up. "Come on, Kale!"

Papa stops me. "Poppie, wait. I really appreciate what you're trying to do. I really do." He exhales a big breath and collapses back against the couch. "But I'm not proposing tomorrow night."

"What?!" I drop to my knees in front of him. "But why? Even if we don't find the ring and the chocolate, I thought you planned to make an incredible dinner and propose?"

Papa looks miserable. "I did. But now I can't." He gestures around him. "No one is here because a couple pipes burst. I have no electricity and no gas. The generator will keep the fridge running, but I have no heat and no stove." He sighs. "Which means no incredible dinner."

No!

I rack my brain. There has to be a way.

I jump up. "You can use my kitchen!"

"Or mine," Kale offers.

Papa shakes his head. "Thank you both, but I'm going to say no. Christmas Eve is a special night to be with your family. I would never think to impose like that."

I open my mouth to disagree, but he stops me.

"Poppie, I have already spoken with Miss Sweettarte and canceled our date. End of discussion."

I stand there stunned. I can't believe he's not going to do it. He and Miss Sweettarte are perfect for each other, and now they won't get engaged. It's just not right.

Papa nods towards the front window. "I see Berg is here to take you home, but before you go, please promise me again that you won't say a word to anyone." He holds out his pinky. "I need this to be our secret."

Kale and I both pinky-promise. I follow Kale to the door, but when I glance back Papa looks so sad that I run back over and give him a big squeezy hug.

"Thanks, Poppie," he says. "It's all for the best anyway."

I don't agree, but I hug him once more before I walk out the door. As I revolve around, I can see him sitting on the couch, head in his hands.

My heart constricts. Poor Papa Shortdough! His market is where everyone goes to be happy. To sit with friends and drink hot cocoa. To nourish our bodies with sandwiches and cookies. To learn how to cook healthy foods so we can get a first kiss. His market is where *he* makes us happy.

And now Papa is alone, and unhappy.

I won't let this happen. I have to figure out a way to help him. A new plan.

Kale and Berg chat about snowboarding on the ride home, but I'm not listening. I'm desperately grasping for a plan that will make Papa Shortdough happy, get my parents home for Christmas Eve dinner, and put everything back the way it used to be. Before all these changes.

Kale taps me on the arm when we reach his house. "Text me later."

I nod, and hand him my backpack with his Mom's clothes.

I rack my brain all the way down Kale's driveway and all the way up mine, but by the time Berg drives into our garage, I still haven't thought of a good plan. I climb out of Berg's Jeep and trudge up the stairs into the house. I'm so frustrated that even Lucy's kisses don't make me feel better.

Berg walks in behind me and drops his gear on the laundry room floor. "Since we're not waiting for Mom and Dad, want to eat now?"

I shake my head. "I'm not hungry."

I can't eat. I have to figure out a plan.

He holds up a takeout bag. "But I got Chicken Tikka Masala from that new Indian place."

"Chicken Tikka Masala?" That gets my attention. It's one of my favorites. And it does smell heavenly. And now that I think about it, I've been so busy all day that I haven't had any junk food snacks, and I'm starving.

Berg shrugs. "I can try to save you a teeny bite or two." He smirks, and walks into the kitchen.

I follow him. "I think I'll eat with you so I get more than a teaspoon."

Berg pulls out plates and forks while I unload the bag. Since it's just the two of us, we sit on the stools in the kitchen to eat. I open the container of rice, dump a little on my plate, and stab it with my fork to spread it out. And then I stab a few more times just to let out some of my frustration.

When I look up, Berg is staring at me. He picks up the container of rice, peeks into it, and shakes his head. "I can't believe they gave me bad rice after I specifically asked them for good rice."

I snort. And almost laugh.

He grabs the container of Chicken Tikka Masala and holds it out of my reach. "Anything you want to talk about before you take it out on the chicken?"

I sigh. "What do you do when you know something should happen and no matter how hard you try to make it happen, you can't make it happen?"

Berg's eyebrows draw together. "That's super vague. Can you be more specific?"

I shake my head. "No."

"Why?"

"I pinky-promised not to tell."

Berg strokes his chin. "But if I guess, you won't be breaking your promise, right?"

I sit up straighter. "Yeah."

He nods. "Okay, did it happen yet?"

"No."

"Is it about Kale?"

"No."

"Mom and Dad?"

"No."

"The mail lady?"

"No!" I groan and throw my hands in the air. "This isn't working."

Berg shovels some chicken onto his plate and passes me the container. "Maybe the budding PI's can read your mind when they get home."

When they get home. I sigh. It's dinnertime, and Berg and I are eating without our parents. This isn't how dinner is supposed to be. But at least I'm here with Berg. Papa Shortdough doesn't have anyone.

I take my first bite, thinking of Papa. I'm curious if what he taught us about mindful eating works on something other than chocolate, so I will try it out. I chew my bite slowly, really trying to taste and savor all the flavors. Creamy coconut, smoky curry, and cool rice. I moan a little. Wow. He's right. Taking more time to chew makes the flavors explode like happiness in my mouth.

"Like it?" Berg asks around a mouthful.

I nod. "I love it. You?"

He shovels in another bite. "Mmm. It's good."

That's saying something because Berg's not a huge fan of... wait a minute!

"You don't like masala."

He shrugs. "But you do."

I blink. He brought home *my* favorite, not his. Knowing Berg, he probably thought it would make me feel better since Mom and Dad wouldn't be here.

He's a pretty cool brother.

And suddenly, I'm smiling.

My parents aren't here, but I'm having a great dinner with my brother. Someday we'll both be married, and probably live too far away to eat dinner together, but today we're here together. Having dinner.

And then I have a pretty adult revelation.

Christmas Eve is not about *Papa's Triple-Chocolate Cookies*, or engagement rings, or evil ovens, or even Mom and Dad being late for dinner. It's about being together. Being together with the people you love in order to bring light and happiness on one of the darkest days of winter.

And suddenly I have my plan.

Santa Claus *will* be coming to town after all.

CHAPTER 16

Even a Hero Needs Help

Berg and I are watching TV when Mom and Dad come home.

They're still wearing head-to-toe black leather and sporting black hair, except Mom has hers long and loose now and no longer in a fake bob.

"How was your first day of school?" I ask, feeling old, and really weird, asking my parents about school.

Mom's face breaks into a huge grin. "So groovy and wonderful!"

"No, Lambikins." Dad pats her gently on the arm. "PI speak."

Mom nods. She raises one eyebrow and glares at us. "I will find the truth. I will hunt you down," she growls. "I will observe the obvious and eliminate the impossible, and then we will know the truth."

Berg's mouth drops open.

Dad claps.

Mom blushes and grins.

"Oh-kay," I say slowly. "I'm guessing you learned how to talk like private investigators tonight?"

"Oh, do you really think I sound like a PI, Poppie Pop?"

Mom's cheeks glow pink.

Dad lifts her up and twirls her around. "Lamikins, that was even better than Professor Sly!"

Mom giggles and pats his chest. "You do it now! Your turn!" She glances at me. "Ask him how his day at school was!"

I think I should ask if they took loopy lessons, but I'm pretty sure I know the answer to that, so instead I cave and ask him.

"Dad, how was your day?" I cringe, anticipating his PI performance.

Dad draws his eyebrows together. He crouches over like he's got a humpback and curls his top lip under to expose his teeth. "It was productive and profitable, and not for the crooks," he croaks in a voice that sounds like a mix between Yoda and the hobbit guy who can't give up that precious thing.

Dad straightens up, and grins. "How was that?"

"Totally creepy," Berg snickers.

Mom jumps into Dad's arms and kisses him for like five minutes.

I can't find any words. Who are these people who gave birth to me?

Mom finally detaches herself from Dad and starts talking about a professor who lives in his car, but I'm only half-listening. I'm trying to figure out how to ask them to help with my plan. I'm afraid they'll say no because I can't tell them any details, but I really need them to say yes for my plan to work.

"I just can't wait to start practicing what we learn," Mom gushes.

I take a deep breath. It's now or never. "How about starting tomorrow?"

One of Dad's eyebrows go up. "What do you mean?"

I have to make this good. Something they can't refuse. "I just happen to know someone who needs a private investigator," I reveal.

"Really?!" Dad asks excitedly. "Who?"

I give them a toothy grin. "Me."

Dad looks confused. "You? Why do you need a PI?"

"I need your help with something, but I can't tell you why."

Dad rubs his hands together. "Okay. Give us all the details!"

I shake my head. "That's just it. I can't."

Mom arches an eyebrow. "You can't?"

"I made a pinky-promise."

Dad nods. "Even PI's don't break a pinky-promise. It's the ultimate word of honor."

I remember what Berg said earlier. "I don't suppose you learned to read minds today?"

Dad shakes his head. "That may be in week three." He taps his chin. "Let me see. What can you tell us without breaking your pinky promise?"

I think for a moment. "Well, I need to have Kale and some kids from *Yum Yum* over tomorrow during the day to help me cook. And I want Papa Shortdough and Miss Sweettarte to join us for Christmas Eve dinner." I shift in my stool. "And I really want you two at Christmas Eve dinner, too. I understand about school, so just tell me when you'll be home and we'll eat then. No matter how late it is." I'm a little embarrassed to seem so needy, but it's really important to me that they're here, so I have to speak up and tell them.

Mom and Dad share a look. I'm not sure how they communicate like that, but they told me once that after 20 years of marriage they just can. It sounds freaky to me. And maybe a little cool.

Mom walks over, puts her arm around me, and grins. "Of course, we'll be here."

"After PI school ends?"

She waves off my question. "Nope. Tomorrow we'll be here at whatever time you need us. Dad and I already decided there's no way we're missing your Christmas Eve dinner."

My heart soars. "Really?"

Mom smiles. "Yes! It's Christmas Eve. And nothing is more

important than being together." She chuckles. "Even hippy PI's know that."

I jump off my stool and squeeze her in a hug. "This is going to be the best Christmas Eve ever!" I turn around, and grin at Berg. "Can the greatest brother in the world give me and my friends a few rides tomorrow?"

Berg bows. "Greatest brother at your service."

I fist punch the air. "This is going to be so sweet!" I inhale a deep breath. "I just hope my plan will work."

Mom rubs her chin like she does when she's deep in thought. "Does your plan have all four components of the hero's journey?"

I give her a funny look. "The what?"

Mom explains. "Well, tonight they said successful plans always follow a hero's journey."

"Seriously?" I'm dumbfounded. "What does being a PI have to do with that?"

"A lot!" Mom says. "A PI has to plan who, what, where, why and when. I guess there have been tons of books written about it."

Dad pipes up. "You have this secret plan, Poppie, so you're the hero."

I blink. "Well, I wouldn't call myself a... hero. More like a meddler."

Mom waves me off. "Oh, come on, don't be modest. I bet you are the hero in this plan. You're the one making it all work." Her eyes grow wide. "And since you can't tell us any details, we can help you be certain you have all the hero components for your plan to work."

"Um, okay." It's worth a try.

Mom claps her hands together. "Okay! Well, first the Hero has to have an Enemy."

An enemy? Nick. Tiffany. Maybe Papa Shortdough when he realizes what I'm doing. "Okay. Check."

Mom nods. "Then the hero has to have a good Sidekick. Someone loyal."

Definitely Kale. But I also need Berg. And Clea, Li and Nacho.

"Can the Hero have more than one Sidekick?" I ask.

Dad nods. "Sure," he says. "Look at those books where the evil guy had a snake and that ferret guy and all those eaters of death guys."

I don't think the evil guy was the hero in that book… but moving on.

"Is that it?" I ask.

"The Hero must overcome a Major Hurdle," Mom says.

Losing twenty pounds so I can get my first kiss is a major hurdle, but that's another plan. This plan is for Papa.

"A Major Hurdle?" I grin. "That's where my amazing parents come in."

Mom looks thoughtful. "I don't think being here for your dinner qualifies as a Major Hurdle."

"Being here for dinner is not the hurdle." I explain. "I need you to get Papa Shortdough here tomorrow."

Dad grunts like I insulted him. "No problem. We don't even need to be PI's to do that."

I make a face. "I think you may have to."

"Why?"

"Because you have to get him to our house without telling him where he's going or why."

Dad raises his eyebrows at Mom. "Deception."

She claps her hands eagerly. "I think we get extra credit for deception!"

Dad smiles at me. "We'll do it."

I sigh with relief. That was easy.

"What's the last component of this journey thing?" Berg asks.

Mom grins. "The Reward, of course!"

I think about that. The Reward. That would be when Papa Shortdough is happy again. And we're all together on Christmas Eve.

Which will only happen if my plan actually works.

Here's hoping for a holly jolly Christmas.

CHAPTER 17

Everyone is Ready to Help!

I wake up the next morning, bursting with elation, anticipation... and a whopping big dose of anxiety.

It's Christmas Eve. Today's our last *Yum Yum* cooking class, and afterwards I need to convince the group to help me.

All I want for Christmas is for my plan to succeed.

I shrug into my orangesicle jacket, and head down the driveway to meet Kale. The sky is vibrant blue. It's bright and sunny, and there's a foot of new snow blanketing the ground, making everything sparkle like a huge glittering ornament.

Kale is waiting for me at our mailboxes.

"Merry Christmas Eve!" he sings out.

"Merry Christmas Eve to you, too!" I unzip my jacket to show him my shirt. It has a picture of a floppy-eared puppy with soulful eyes holding a destroyed shoe in its mouth. The bubble caption above reads:

Dear Santa, does naughty count if you do it very, very nicely?

Kale grins. "We must have been thinking the same thing this morning." He unzips his neon green jacket and pulls out his tie. It's sparkling red with white writing on it that reads:

Dear Santa, I've been very good.
No matter what anyone else says!

I laugh. "We definitely were."

We start walking towards main street, our boots leaving fresh tracks in the snow. I told Kale my plan last night and he seemed okay with it. But I wonder if this morning he's having second thoughts. I know I expect him to always go along with my plans, but he's my best friend and I would never want him to do something he really doesn't want to do.

I punch the walk button at the stoplight. "You know you can still back out."

He shakes his head. "And leave all this sneaking around to you? No way. I'm totally in." He gives me a playful shove. "You worried?"

I snort. "Let's see. I've concocted a devious plan that uses my PI-in-training parents to deceive Papa Shortdough and do something he told me not to do. Why would I be worried? I'm pretty sure Santa is already moving my name to the naughty list as we speak."

Kale links his arm through mine as we walk across the street. "I doubt that. Your plan is actually very caring and sweet."

I frown. "Except that Papa Shortdough may hate me forever."

Kale shrugs. "Maybe. But I highly doubt it." He looks at me with a twinkle in his eye. "Because who can be mad at you when you are so *very, very nice*?"

I chuckle. I sure am lucky to have Kale as a best friend *and* a sidekick.

The clock outside Butte Mountain Resort chimes once at nine-thirty. Skiers and riders are already streaming down the slopes, but Main Street is still fairly quiet. The last-minute holiday shoppers must still be sleeping.

I stop Kale when we reach Papa's Market. "Let's wait out here so we can catch Clea before she goes in."

Kale points to the big CLOSED sign on the market's window. "Looks like Papa's not open yet anyway."

I try to push the revolving door. It doesn't budge. I frown.

"That's weird. He's usually opens at seven." I press my face up to the glass and peer inside.

Kale presses his face up to the glass next to me. "Maybe he's opening late because it's Christmas Eve?"

"What are you two doing?" Tiffany's voice shrills behind us, startling me so bad that I bang my nose on the glass.

I turn around, rubbing my shiny red nose. Tiffany is decked out in a white sweater dress adorned with every glittering crystal ever made. She is standing with one hand on her hip and one hand holding Nick's arm.

Tiffany notices the sign and scrunches up her nose. "Closed? On Christmas Eve? Why would Papa Shortdough do that?"

"Looks like you can ask him yourself," Kale replies as Papa Shortdough spins out of the revolving door to join us.

"Good morning, everyone." He tries to smile, but the corners of his mouth look too tired to rise, and instead of his food-splattered apron, he's wearing a ski hat and a dark blue ski jacket.

Tiffany points to the sign. "Why are you closed?"

Papa shades his eyes from the blinding glitz shooting off Tiffany's outfit. "Because my power is still out." He motions to the door. "Please come inside until the others arrive."

Tiffany struts into the revolving door with Nick following her. Kale and I hang behind. I still need to talk to Clea alone.

Papa motions again to the door. "Come on, you two. Let's talk inside."

We can't tell him why we want to stay outside, so we follow him into the market. After standing in the warm sun, it feels cold and damp inside, mimicking Papa's mood. I miss his crinkly smile, and his laugh, and his thumb war prowess. I hope what I'm about to do will make him happy again, and not make his gloomy mood worse!

"Might as well sit down while we wait," Papa mutters, but then adds, "Ah, there they are."

He motions Clea, Li, and Nacho into the market. Clea is

wearing a puffy parka today, and Nacho and Li are wearing matching red-and-blue Barcelona fútbol jackets.

Li nods to the CLOSED sign in the window, making her red Santa earrings dance. "Want me to flip that to OPEN?"

Papa shakes his head. "No, I have to stay closed today. I'm sorry I couldn't save you all a trip over here. I thought everything would be back to normal this morning but my power is still out and one of the busted pipes created quite a mess in the kitchen. I'm sorry, but I'm going to have to reschedule our class until after Christmas when everything is cleaned up."

"Maybe we can help you clean?" Kale offers.

There's a chorus of 'Yes!' and 'Yeah!' and 'Good idea!' coming from everyone, except Tiffany, who's suddenly super interested in her furry, white boots.

Papa holds his hands up in front of him. "Thank you, but my insurance company is sending someone over to take care of it." He tries to smile but it doesn't reach the dark bags under his eyes. "I want to thank all of you for the hard work you've put in these last two days. It's been fun teaching you. Now go and enjoy your Christmas Eve. I'll email you when we can make up our last class."

Tiffany immediately says goodbye and leaves, tugging Nick out with her.

I intercept Clea as she's walking over to Papa. "Do you have the recipes?" I whisper.

Clea nods.

"Good. Don't give them to Papa. I have an idea."

Clea looks skeptical, but nods. "Okay."

Li joins us. "This is such a bummer. I feel so bad for Papa."

"I do, too," I agree. "I have a plan to help Papa feel better, but it has to be a surprise to him. If you guys are free today I could really use your help."

"I'm free all day," Li says.

"Me, too," adds Clea.

I grin. "Great! Let's meet over at the resort as soon as we leave here."

Li nods. "You got it. Want me to bring Nacho?"

"Yes! That would be great."

I turn to Clea. "Are you in?"

Since her black hair is back in a long braid today, I can see her cocoa eyes smile before she does. "You bet. I'll be there."

The three of us join Kale and Nacho who are talking to Papa. He looks miserable.

"I'm so sorry about all this," Papa says. "This is not the way I thought Christmas Eve would end up, but I guess we'll just have to make the best of it."

We all take turns giving him hugs. Clea, Li and Nacho say their goodbyes and walk out together, but Kale and I linger for another moment.

Papa tugs one of my braids. "Poppie, I know you'll make your family a fantastic Christmas Eve dinner. You just have to believe in yourself." He winks at me. "You know I do."

My heart soars. Even when he feels at his worst, he's still trying to make me happy and confident. This is why my plan just has to work!

I throw my arms around him in a hug. "Thanks, Papa."

He holds onto me and pulls Kale into our hug. "I'm lucky to have you two great kids in my life." He smiles, and this time his eyes crinkle like he means it. "Have a very happy Christmas." He releases us from the hug and gently pushes us towards the door. "Now get out of here," he barks, but keeps his smile bright as he says it.

As we head over to the revolving door, I whisper to Kale. "I think this calls for a Christmas song."

He nods, the green spikes on his hat waving in agreement.

We both jump into the same opening and revolve around and around, singing *We wish you a Merry Christmas* loud and shrieky and with all our love poured into it. The last thing I see before I tumble out onto the sidewalk is Papa Shortdough's huge smile. I hope to see it again later after he realizes what I did.

We dash across the street to the resort and find Clea, Li, and Nacho sitting in front of the big window that looks out onto the slopes.

Li waves us over. "Yo," she says. "So, what's the plan?"

I explain every part of my plan that I can, leaving out anything that would break my pinky-promise to Papa.

"I'm in!" Li says, barely a second after I finish talking. "I'd do anything for Papa Shortdough!"

"Me, too!" Clea adds. "I just need to figure out a ride."

Nacho nods his head. "Same for me."

"I'm pretty sure my mom can pick us all up later," Li offers. "I just need to call her."

I clap my hands together. "You guys are the best! Figure out your rides, and we'll meet out front in five minutes."

While they call their parents, Kale wanders over to look at the new snowboards, and I walk up to the window, smiling at the skiers and riders whipping down the slopes.

"It'll never work," a voice grunts behind me.

I whip my head around to find Nick right behind me. Surprisingly, he's not dressed in his typical black but is wearing a white sweater and jeans. Even more surprising is that he looks very cute in it. The white brings out the gold flecks in his chocolaty brown eyes.

Wait a minute.

I frown. "What do you mean it'll never work?"

He shrugs. "Your plan. It won't work."

I gasp. "What plan?"

He rolls his eyes. "The one you were just telling your friends about."

"You were eavesdropping!" I ball my hands into fists. I want to slug him! If he tells Papa Shortdough, it could ruin everything!

He sighs. "I just happened to be nearby, heard Papa Shortdough's name, and wanted to be certain no one was messing with him." He chuckles. "Although, he may not be very happy with what you're planning."

I narrow my eyes. "If you say a word to Papa, I'll tell everyone about the socks."

He gawks at me as if I have a ski sticking out of my head. "The socks?"

"Yeah!" I smirk. "The ones you don't want anyone to know you collect."

His cheeks actually turn a bit pink. "Whatevs. I wasn't going to snitch on you. I was just wondering if my Nams knows she's coming?"

I slap my forehead. I never figured that part out.

He grunts. "I didn't think so. Right now she has plans with me tonight." He looks down at the ground. "I can help get her there if you want."

My eyes almost pop out of my head. "You want to help?"

He shrugs. "My Nams deserves happiness as much as anyone else."

I blink. Well, that was sweet. But can I trust him? What if he's just playing with me and ruins my entire plan? I did have him pegged as the enemy.

I groan inside. Trust or not, I need his help.

I put my hands on my hips. "Okay, but she can't know why, or where, or what's going on."

He nods. "Got it." He tugs his black hat lower on his forehead, then stares right at me. "This is nice what you're doing. Really nice." His full lips turn up into what looks like an embarrassed smile. He opens his mouth to say something, but then closes it and shrugs. "I knew... well... what I meant was...you're a really nice girl, and I like that about you."

I'm so confused. What is happening?

He Clears his throat. "Anyway, I'll get Nams there." He glances around to make sure no one is listening before whispering, "And let's just keep this helping thing between you and me. Could be bad for my reputation." Then he grins at me and walks away.

I'm in shock. What just happened? Does Nick Sweettarte actually have a heart? And did he say he liked me?

My heart starts beating very fast.

No, wait. Slow down there huge one. He didn't say he

liked *me*. I'm too fat to have a cute boy like me. He said he liked that I was nice. That's a big difference.

I just hope he gets her to my house without being run over by a reindeer.

CHAPTER 18

Miss Sweettarte Almost Finds Out

Since Papa's Market is closed, we head over to the grocery in the neighboring town of Peak. There are no open parking spots so Berg drops us off in front. We make plans to meet him in twenty minutes. I figure with five of us shopping that should give us plenty of time.

Clea is still scribbling out a grocery list, so Nacho and Li each grab a shoulder and steer her into the store. Kale and I head over to grab a cart.

It's so busy that there are only two left. I grab one and pull it, expecting it to release from the other, but it doesn't budge. I try again to pry them apart, but no luck. They're as stuck as gum in frizzy hair.

Kale Clears his throat. "Need some help?"

"Yeah." I get a firm grip on the handle. "You pull that one from the back."

He nods and grabs hold.

"On three. One, two, three!"

I pull the front. He pulls the back. And THWAAAP they release, and I go flying backwards, taking the cart with me. I stumble over my feet as the cart fights hard to run me over, but I regain my balance and stand up. I push the cart towards Kale, only to be rewarded with a loud *SCREE, SCREE, SCREE* every time the wheel turns.

I stop. I push it forward again. *SCREE, SCREE, SCREE*

Kale is bent over, laughing so hard he can barely talk. "Other... one?"

I raise an eyebrow. "I'm thinking that would be swell."

We grab the other cart and meet up with the others.

"What's first on the list?" I ask Clea.

She points to the produce section in front of us. "Apples."

Everyone follows Clea to the apples. I'm maneuvering the cart closer when I see Miss Sweettarte enter the store.

I panic. She can't see us shopping here!

"Everyone hide!" I hiss and duck down behind the apple bin.

Kale drops down beside me. "What's going on?" he whispers.

"Miss Sweettarte just walked in," I yelp.

Nacho is squatting on the other side of me. "Why we not want her to see us?"

I don't know how to answer him. That was the part I couldn't tell them. Kale and I exchange looks.

"What's going on?" I hear Li whisper to Nacho.

"Miss Sweettarte is here," he whispers back.

"Oh, I love her," Li gushes. "She's always so smiley."

"Poppie says we hide from her," Nacho says uncertainly.

"Why?" Li asks.

Nacho shrugs and looks at me.

I ignore him, and look at Kale. "I'm going to check out where she is."

Kale nods.

I turn back to Nacho. "Tell everyone to stay down."

He nods and whispers to Li, who then whispers to Clea.

I slowly stand up. I stay low and keep my face hidden by the towering piles of apples. I scan the front of the store but can't find her. I lean a little left. She's not by the lettuce or the mushrooms. I lean a little right, but the bin of apples is still blocking my view. I lean a little farther... Oops! That was too far. I throw my arms out, trying to stop my fall, but all I grab are slippery apples. I tumble backwards and throw my hands up to protect my face while a deluge of apples plop plop plop all around me.

"Goodness gracious! Poppie? Is that you? Are you all right, darlin'?"

I peek through my hands and see Miss Sweettarte staring down at me. I manage a wave. "Hi, Miss Sweettarte," I croak.

Her eyebrows knit together. I can see her brain trying to figure out why I'm lying on the floor, covered in apples, surrounded by four, crouching kids. Her pink-lips pull into a thin line.

"What *are* y'all doin'?"

Kale stands up. "Hide and seek!" He points at me. "And Poppie found us!"

A grocery clerk rushes over. His expression darkens when he sees all the apples on the floor. "What in the world happened here?" he shrieks.

Miss Sweettarte puts her hands on her hips. "Now, don't get a burr in your saddle, young man. It's just a few apples. That's no reason to holler like that."

The clerk tears his eyes away from the apple fiesta on the floor and his eyebrows pop up. "Oh, Miss Sweettarte...hello, ma'am!"

Have I mentioned that everyone adores her?

Miss Sweettarte parts her lips into a heart-melting grin and puts her hand on the clerk's arm. "Oh, my darlin' boy, I think this was all my fault." She pouts out her bottom lip. "I'm so sorry, but I scared the poor dears and all your beautiful apples jumped for freedom."

The clerk smiles and pats her hand. "It's quite okay, Miss Sweettarte. Like you said, it's just a few apples."

I'm flabbergasted at her effect on people. All she has to do is smile and say a few words, and she magically transforms people from angry to happy. She's truly special. I hope my plan works so we can make her happy, too.

Miss Sweettarte links her arm through the clerk's arm. She winks at me before she starts leading him away from us. "I know you must be very busy today, darlin', so don't you worry your pretty head about this. I'll make sure they clean this up faster than a hot knife through butter." I can't hear the rest of their conversation, but the clerk gives her a toothy grin before he hurries off. She walks back over to us, and extends her arms. "Ta Da!"

I grin. "You're amazing!"

She chuckles. "Not at all, darlin'. I just learned long ago that sugar is sweeter than vinegar." She glances at the apples. "Now about this?"

"Oh, don't worry, ma'am," I assure her. "I'll clean them up. Thanks again for your help."

She nods.

I wait for her to leave, but she doesn't.

"So... you're shopping?" I say to fill the silence. I realize too late what I just asked. Papa Shortdough canceled their dinner and now she has to find something else to eat tonight. I give myself a mental head slap.

Miss Sweettarte's smile fades. I think I see tears spring to her eyes, but she looks away and when she looks back at me, they're gone.

"Just a last minute need for some groceries." She hesitates like she wants to say more, but then waves her hand like it isn't important. "Well, I must skedaddle," she insists. "Merry Christmas Eve to all of y'all. Ta ta."

I sure hope what we have planned later will cheer her up. I glance at my watch. "We have to meet my brother in fifteen minutes. I'll clean this up. You guys start grabbing the other stuff we need."

"I'll help Poppie," Kale offers.

Clea glances at her list, and then takes charge. "Okay. Li, please get carrots. Nacho, pomegranate seeds. And I'll get the spinach." She grabs my discarded cart, and the three of them disperse across the produce section.

Kale and I start picking up apples and putting them in a bag. I figure my little tumble probably bruised them, so I should buy them. Some of them may still work in our recipe, but if not, I'll just give them to Miss Sweettarte's horses as a Christmas treat.

"I can't believe no one said anything about my plan," I whisper to Kale as I put two really bruised apples into the bag. I must have fallen on top of them.

"I told them not to."

I widen my eyes. "Did you tell them why?"

Kale looks like I just slapped him. "No way! You know I would never break a pinky promise! I just said in case Miss Sweettarte sees Papa today we better not to mention your plan to her."

I grin. "Very smart thinking, dude."

He grins back, and ties the first full bag closed with a flourish.

We pick up the rest of the apples and find the others shopping a few aisles away. Clea is crossing items off her list while instructing Nacho and Li what to get next. She seems to be in complete control. I think of how far she's come from that shy girl who hid behind her hair on our first day of class. I don't know if it's because she found something she's good at, or if it's just having friends who believe in her, but whatever it is, I'm happy to be a part of it.

We grab the rest of the food with four minutes to spare until we have to meet Berg.

I push the cart up to the checkout. I'm shocked to find a fairly empty line behind a lady wearing a tailored, navy suit. Her groceries are all bagged, and she's just about to pay. I'm congratulating myself on scoring the shortest line on this busy day when I see her pull out a stack of coupons.

She hands them to the clerk. "I spend an hour every morning before work clipping coupons," she says proudly.

I glance at my watch. We only have three minutes until we're supposed to meet Berg. I debate changing lanes, but Clea and I have already emptied our groceries onto the belt. I watch the clerk scan all of the coupons, and then look at my watch. Two minutes left. We should still make it.

But then the lady flutters her hand to her face. "Oh, my, I almost forgot." She throws a red purse as big as a briefcase onto the checkout counter and rummages around in it. "There they are," she announces and pulls out another stack of coupons, way thicker than her first stack.

Clea and I exchange looks.

"This could take a while," I whisper. I shimmy around to the back of the cart where Kale, Li, and Nacho are chatting.

"We are behind the coupon queen of the west," I mutter. "Will someone please go outside and tell Berg we're coming?"

Kale volunteers. As he leaves, Miss Sweettarte walks up to our line. She's carrying a handcart with only a few items in it.

"It's like ticks on a dog in here," she scowls. "Every line except yours is a mile long!" She whistles when she sees our groceries on the belt. "Goodness gracious! That's a load of food. Are y'all having a party tonight?"

I laugh too loud. "Ha! Ha! Ha! A party?" I shake my head. "No. No. Nope."

The belt starts moving. I glance behind me and see the coupon queen is gone and the clerk is scanning our food. I give Li and Nacho a gentle shove toward the front of the basket. "Would you two mind helping Clea bag?" I don't mean to be bossy, but I'm so afraid they're going to say something about my plan. I turn back to Miss Sweettarte. "Well, I better help them, but I hope you have a very Merry Christmas."

"Merry Christmas to you, too, darlin' Poppie." She tries to smile but looks so sad and heartbroken, like the only dog left at the pound on Christmas Eve, that I almost tell her everything.

But I don't.

I just give her a squeezy hug, and hope deep in my heart that her grandson keeps his promise.

Or it's going to be a very silent night.

CHAPTER 19

The Yum Yum Club

Almost every inch of my kitchen counter is covered with food. It looks like the grocery store relocated to my house, and then exploded. Even the ceramic chicken that holds Lucy's treats is crushed against the wall, gasping for air.

Kale plops the last bag on the counter and looks at me. "Where do we start, mighty planner?"

I suddenly panic. Where *do* we start? There are too many groceries, too much to do, and only two hours to do it. This is never going to work.

Clea must see the panic in my eyes. She pulls out the recipes and hands them to me. "I can help you. While the recipes were printing last night, I kind of worked out the timing in case Papa wanted us to make the meal in class."

I exhale a huge breath. "Sweet." I get everyone's attention. "I would like to nominate Clea as our Head Chef."

Li's hand shoots up. "I second that."

Kale nods. "I third it."

Nacho grins. "Then I give it a four."

"Clea..." I lean towards her. "What's your middle name?"

She blushes slightly. "Margaret."

I roll the recipes up to look like a sword and gently tap

each of her shoulders. "Clea Margaret, I appoint you Head Chef!"

She smiles so wide you'd think it was her birthday. She curtsies. "Thank you."

I motion to the mess of groceries. "You're in charge now, girlfriend. Tell us what to do."

Her eyes widen a little, and I wonder if she's panicking, but then she rubs her hands together. "Let's start cooking."

Clea gives each of us a job, and soon the kitchen counter doesn't seem unorganized and chaotic. It seems lively and bustling, and even a bit orderly, which is just how I like it.

Li and Nacho are mixing dough for the rolls. Kale is toasting walnuts for the salad. I'm making batter for the chocolate cupcakes. And Clea is carefully spreading yogurt on the chicken breasts, her tongue sticking out of the corner of her mouth in concentration.

Lucy walks into the kitchen, sits right on Clea's foot and barks. Clea jumps a little. Lucy barks again.

I laugh. "I think she wants the chicken." I shake my head at Lucy. "No, silly girl, it's still raw."

Clea laughs. She bends over to pet Lucy and wins a kiss on her cheek. She giggles. "Maybe Poppie will save you a bite." She looks questioningly at me.

I nod, but before I can say anything, Li claps her hands.

"Attention, please! Or *atención,* for our Spanish friend." She winks at Nacho. "I just wanted to thank all of you. I've loved learning to cook the last couple days with Papa Shortdough and I've loved getting to know all of you." She grins, and with a devilish gleam in her eye, she holds up her flour-covered hands. "So, it is my honor to officially induct everyone into *The Yum Yum Club!*"

Nacho is standing next to her and before he can react, Li slaps his back, leaving a pure white handprint on his red-and-blue jersey. "Nacho is now officially a member of *The Yum Yum Club!*" she proclaims.

He looks shocked for a second, and then laughs. "I am honor!"

She zips over to Clea next, branding her with a flour handprint. "Clea is now officially a member of *The Yum Yum Club!*"

Clea throws her arms around Li and hugs her. A look of surprise crosses Li's face but she hugs her back. "And, officially, my friend," Li declares. Clea beams.

Li turns to Kale and holds up her palms. "Your turn," she chuckles.

Kale dashes around the counter but Li catches him and smacks a handprint right in the middle of his tie. "Kale is now officially a member of *The Yum Yum Club!*"

Kale looks down at his tie and grins. "Better than a snowball fight," he laughs.

Li looks at me with a devilish grin. "Now, for the gal with the plan. The gal who got us all together." She waggles her eyebrows. "Everyone has to induct her!"

They all cover their hands with the flour left on the counter and hold up their palms, chanting *"Yum Yum"* as they surround me in a circle. It's weird and goofy, but I'm smiling so wide and my heart is bursting with so much happiness that it's taking my breath away. I'm so happy I met all of them at Papa's class.

We're all laughing so hard as they slap flour handprints all over me that we don't even notice Berg walk into the kitchen.

"I can see the cooking is going well," he laughs.

I grin. "*The Yum Yum Club* has got it under control."

"Well, good because Mom just called."

My palms grow sweaty. "With good or bad news?"

He winks. "Good! She said everything is going according to your plan."

I exhale. Whew.

"And they'll be here in about 30 minutes," he adds.

"What?!"

I glance at the clock. Oh no. It's already four o'clock! Where did the time go? We're nowhere near ready and there's flour everywhere.

I run my hands along my braids, and start pacing. "We still

have to cook the cupcakes, chicken and carrots, toss the salad, set the table, and cook the rolls." I grab the top of my head because I'm pretty sure my brain is about to explode. "The five of us will never get it all done!"

"Six," Berg says.

I stare at him.

He points to himself. "Six."

I see his confident smile and feel my heartbeat slow a bit. I glance around the room. Everyone is staring at me, waiting to see what I decide. Waiting to see if we can do it. Waiting for my decision.

"We can do it," Clea whispers.

Kale nods in agreement. Li gives me a thumbs up, and Nacho grins.

Goosebumps rise on my skin. They're right. We can do it. For Papa Shortdough, we can do anything.

I grin. "Let's get back to work then!"

Everyone returns to their jobs, and Clea asks Berg to set the table. Lucy even tries to help by licking every bit of flour off the floor that she can.

I finish spooning out the batter and put the cupcakes in the oven. When Clea assigned me dessert, I wanted to say no because it involved something I could burn. But I knew I needed to try again. Besides, I'm not going to let the oven ruin this. Instead of setting a timer, I have a new plan. I'm just going to stand here and wait until they smell done.

I glare at the oven, and raise my eyebrows. "I will win this time," I whisper.

I sniff the air. Nope. Not done yet.

I wait.

And I wait.

Ugh! This is taking forever!

I eye the clock, and sigh. Only two minutes have passed! I can't just stand here. I'm wasting time. I should be doing something else to get ready.

I scan the kitchen. Clea is shredding cheese. Nacho and Li

are shaping rolls out of dough and placing them on a tray. Kale is tossing spinach into a bowl with one hand, and trying to chop walnuts with the other.

"Hey, Kale," I yell over, "Need some help?"

"That'd be great," he answers without looking up.

I'm sure I can still smell the cupcakes while I chop walnuts, but just in case, I set the timer on the oven. Better safe than burned.

I hurry over to Kale. He hands me the knife and shoots me a look of relief.

"Thanks. Just toss them on top of the spinach. I'm going to whip up the dressing."

I cut the walnuts and add them to his salad. I'm headed back over to check on my cupcakes when Li squeals.

"Look everyone, it's snowing!"

And just like that, I forget all about the timer, my cupcakes, and the cursed oven.

Let it snow. Let it snow. Let it snow.

CHAPTER 20

You Gotta Know How to Tweak

We're standing by my front window, watching big, fluffy snowflakes float and dance through the trees and fall gently to the ground.

"I like seeing this," Nacho murmurs as he presses his nose to the window. "It only snow in Barcelona maybe one a year."

Li claps excitedly, and when she grins I see a glimpse of what she probably looked like as a little girl. "I hope it snows all night long and we wake up to a white Christmas!"

Kale closes his eyes and crosses his fingers. "And if Santa comes through, I'll be riding my new board tomorrow in knee-deep, fresh powder!"

Li points to a black SUV coming up the driveway. "There's my dad." A panicked look crosses her face. "Wait! Clea, did we finish everything?"

Clea nods, and grins. "Yes, we did."

Li high fives her. "Oh yeah! Never underestimate what *The Yum Yum…*," she pauses. "What's that?"

We all listen. It's a faint, almost musical *ding… ding… ding.* It sounds like… OH NO!

I sprint into the kitchen, yank open the oven, and a cloud of smoke engulfs me. I bravely fight my way through the haze and rescue the cupcakes. But when I set them on the counter I realize all is lost.

They're burned.

Scorched.

Charred.

Ruined.

I'm so embarrassed that I can't even look anyone in the eye. I hang my head. "I'm so sorry. I totally fried them."

Clea pats my arm. "That's okay. We'll just make new ones." She turns to Li. "Can your dad wait five minutes? If we all work together..."

I interrupt her. "We can't." I shake my head. "We're out of cocoa."

"That's okay," Kale says. "You guys start on the batter, and I'll get Berg to run me to the store. We'll be back in fifteen minutes."

I glance at the clock. It's already four-thirty. Mom and Dad – and hopefully Papa Shortdough- will be here any minute.

I shake my head. "There's not enough time." I slump onto the stool and drop my forehead onto the counter. "It's official," my lips mumble into the granite. "I don't deserve to be in *The Yum Yum Club*. Poppie Pie Sunshine Wellington really, truly *can't* cook."

Kale gently pulls up my head. "Come on, Poppie. You know that's not true." He shrugs. "So, you burned something. Who cares! *You* had the plan. *You* got us all together. *You* are as much a part of this club as the rest of us. We wouldn't even be here if it weren't for you and your plan!"

"He's right," Clea says. "We're all here cooking together because of you."

Li slaps me on the back. "You made us into *The Yum Yum Club!*"

Nacho points to the blackened cupcakes. "Poppie, I try one?"

I snort. "Only if you want to poison yourself."

He shakes his head. "I eat many foods with my host family that look worse. I think your cupcakes will not be poison."

I wave my hand. "Help yourself."

Nacho unwraps the cupcake and sets it on a napkin. He leans closer, examines it from every angle, then gently peels off the burned top and sets it aside. Using a sharp knife, he cuts a small piece off the remaining cupcake and pops it into his mouth.

I wait for him to gag and spit it out like Lucy did with my blackened cookies, but instead his face breaks into a huge grin. "Is good!" He cuts another piece and tries to hand it to me. "You try!"

I hold up my hands to protect myself from the charred chocolate. "There's no way that could be good. It's burnt!"

Li grabs the piece from Nacho, pops it into her mouth and chews. I flinch, expecting a horror movie face, but she surprises me. Her eyes light up and she grins. "He's right, Poppie. It is good. Really good!"

Kale and Clea each grab a piece.

Kale chews, and doesn't even swallow before he declares. "It's de-thicious!"

I roll my eyes.

Clea swallows her bite and her eyes twinkle. "They're really not ruined, Poppie. They're perfect!" She holds a piece out to me. "Just try one."

I sigh. "Fine." I take the piece, debate holding my nose, but instead just toss it into my mouth and take my punishment. The cupcake is still warm and dense like a brownie. And I can't believe it, but they're right. It's good. The chocolate now has a smoky richness that reminds me of eating s'mores around a campfire.

Kale swallows his bite. "If Papa were here, he'd tell you that you didn't burn them, you just tweaked them. And then he'd wink at you and tell you what a great chef you are." He pauses to flex his muscles and winks at me, trying to imitate Papa.

I laugh at Kale's impression, but what he said reminds me of what Papa told me after I burned the pancakes. He said when everything doesn't go as planned, the tweaks you make are what make the recipe - and life! – so sweet.

So… I guess it's time for some tweaking.

"Okay then," I nod my head. "Change of plan. We toss the tops, cut the cupcakes into pieces, and…" I pause, debating what else to do.

"You have any ice cream?" Kale asks.

"Yes!" Li says excitedly. "They'd be awesome with ice cream!"

"And berries?" Clea offers.

"Or bananas?" Nacho adds.

I nod, suddenly really excited about this new dessert. "All these ideas are so sweet!" I rush over and yank open the freezer. "Ice cream!" I scream. "And it's even vanilla."

Clea grins. "Then let's cut the cupcakes."

I pull out raspberries and bananas, and set them on the counter. "I'd love your help, but isn't Li's dad waiting outside to take you all home?"

Li waves her hand. "Don't worry. I just texted him that we'd be a few more minutes, and he said no problemo."

I grin. "Sweet. Thanks."

As we work together to make the new dessert, I realize how lucky I am that my plan went wonky. I burned something, but with the help of my friends, I didn't give up. Instead, they're helping me tweak it into something totally different that will be totally delicious. A mound of chocolate cake bites topped with ice cream, raspberries and bananas. It's a smoky sundae that will be a perfect Christmas Eve dessert.

I clap my hands. "We should call these *Chocolate Chimney Cupcakes* in honor of Santa!"

"I love it!" Li exclaims.

Kale nods. "Perfect tribute to the big guy."

The next few minutes are a blur as we finish up. Li and Nacho head for the door, while Clea puts the chicken in the oven and hands me the instructions.

"Just in case, I set the timer to go off a little early," she says with a smile.

I hug her. "You're the absolute best, you know that, right?"

The old, shy Clea makes a reappearance as she blushes and ducks her head. "Aw, thanks," she murmurs. "I'm really happy to have you as a friend, Poppie."

I grin. "I'm really happy you're my friend, Clea."

We hug each other one more time before she hurries out the door and climbs into the SUV with Li and Nacho.

I yell out to all of them. "Thanks *Yum Yum Club*! I couldn't have done it without you!"

They all wave back as they drive away.

I close the door and join Kale back in the kitchen. I'm about to thank him for all his hard work when I hear the garage door open.

My stomach flip-flops. "They're here!" I cry.

Kale grins. "It's okay. We're all ready."

I look around the kitchen and take a quick inventory. He's right. The sides are ready. The dessert is tweaked. The chicken is in the oven, smelling delicious. I exhale a deep breath. This is going to work.

Or so I believe for a full three seconds before Mom and Dad walk into the kitchen.

Alone.

Without Papa Shortdough.

My face falls. "Where's Papa? Could you not convince him? Is he not coming?" I can't get the words out fast enough. "All this work! All this preparation! All for nothing."

Dad holds up his hand. "Poppie, calm down. He's here."

"Where? Where is he?" I have a horrible thought. "You didn't tell him did you? Is he so mad that he won't even come inside?"

Mom shakes her head. "Oh, no, we didn't tell him." Her face turns grim as she purses her lips in a tight line. "He's in the car. We thought he may be safer in there until we figure out..." She looks over at Dad and trails off.

Uh oh.

"Figure out what?"

Neither of them answers me.

I feel a bubble of panic in my chest. My voice comes out in a high-pitched, I'm-about-to-lose-it squeal. "What do you need to figure out?"

Dad's face breaks into a crooked smile. "How to un-hypnotize him."

"Huh?" I shake my head. "I think I heard you wrong. You need to what?"

"We need to UN-hypnotize him."

I look over at Mom. "You hypnotized him?"

She nods.

Kale is cracking up. "You hypnotized Papa. This is so awesome!"

Dad smiles "Thanks, bud. It was our first time, and it did seem to go well."

Mom pipes up. "The good news is that he doesn't know where he is." She's using her extra-perky voice, so I know there's bad news coming.

I sigh. "What's the bad news?"

She grimaces. "He doesn't know *who* he is."

Oh, silver bells.

CHAPTER 21

Papa's Not Quite Himself

Mom paces back and forth in the kitchen. "We tried every way we learned to bring him out of it. We snapped our fingers, counted backwards. We even splashed some water on his face." She shakes her head. "Nothing's working."

Berg walks into the kitchen. "What's not working?"

I throw up my hands. "Mom and Dad hypnotized Papa Shortdough, *but* they can't figure out how to un-hypnotize him."

Berg raises his eyebrows and grins. ""You can hypnotize people? So. Cool."

Dad shrugs and Mom smiles shyly.

I crumple onto the stool. "It *would* be cool if they knew how to un-hypnotize people." As soon as the words are out of my mouth, I see Mom's face fall and I regret saying them. I'm about to apologize when the garage door slams and Papa Shortdough walks into the kitchen.

I gasp.

His eyes are glazed and wide-open, kind of like how a cartoon character looks when it's been hit on the head. He's dressed in a gray suit, but has his red tie in his hands.

"Papa," I whisper.

He swings his head in the direction of my voice, stares at me unblinking for a second and then suddenly jumps to life.

"Out of the way," he shouts, never once blinking his eyes. "I'm here to save the day!" He raises his tie over his head and spins it like a lasso. He races across the kitchen, stops in front of the fat, yellow, ceramic chicken holding Lucy's treats, and sticks his head down next to it. "I need your help!" he hisses. He grabs the yellow head, holds it out in front of him, and races past us into the front room, those red chicken lips leading the way.

"Oh, dear," Mom says. She shares a look with Dad. "Maybe we shouldn't have been talking about superheroes on the way over here." They both rush after him.

I jump up to follow them, but screech to a stop in the doorway where they are staring into the front room. Dad puts his finger to his lips and points to Papa who is in deep conversation with the table lamp.

"Traitors with umbrellas can never be trusted!" he's warning the lamp. He nods quickly as if the lamp is talking to him, then spins around a few times before kneeling down beside the coffee table. He wraps his hand around one leg and wiggles his thumb around.

Kale is behind me, peeking around my shoulder. "He's having a thumb war with your coffee table," he whispers, trying to snort back his laughter.

I try not to laugh. I really do. But it's just beyond funny watching Papa in his suit wrestling with the coffee table. I slam my hand over my mouth trying to keep my giggles quiet.

Papa hears us, jumps up onto the couch, and points the chicken head at us. "Aha! Traitors! Do you have umbrellas?"

No one says anything. I see Mom shake her head.

Papa points right at her. "You!" he yells.

She jumps.

He leaps off the couch, marches over to her, and thrusts the chicken head within an inch of her face. He tilts his head from side to side, staring at her without blinking.

Mom's eyes are wide and un-blinking, too, but her lips are

moving, muttering something that sounds like a Chinese food menu.

Papa suddenly tucks the chicken head under his arm, walks over to the couch, and sits down. Mom says some mumbo-jumbo a little louder, and Papa flops sideways onto the couch, cradling the chicken head. Within seconds, he's sound asleep and snoring.

Dad pushes us all back into the kitchen. I plop onto a stool and Kale sits next to me.

Kale apologizes to Dad. "I didn't mean to laugh," he whispers, "but that was hilarious."

I think I see Dad smile, but it quickly disappears when he sees the look on my face.

"Can you get him back to his normal self?" I plead.

Dad nods. "We'll find a way. Don't worry."

"But I am worried!" I try to keep my voice down. "We have exactly NO minutes until I need Papa to be himself or my plan will never work." I gesture to the food surrounding us. "And all of this will be for nothing."

Mom walks into the kitchen with her lips in a tight line. I raise my eyebrows hopefully. She shakes her head.

I moan. "But it seemed like he was listening to you."

She nods. "He did seem to be responding to the Great Wall technique, but to be honest," she pauses and we can all hear Papa snoring as loud as a buzzsaw. She grimaces. "I'm afraid I may have hypnotized him even more."

I suddenly feel light-headed. "More?"

Mom nods.

DING DONG

Mom's eyebrows draw together. "Who's that?"

I groan. "I'll take care of it. Please keep working on Papa."

I jump off my stool, tiptoe past Papa, and reach the door just as the doorbell chimes again.

DING DONG

I open the door a tiny crack, expecting to see Miss Sweettarte and Nick and somehow convince them to leave, but instead I'm face to face with glossy hair and a scowl.

It's Tiffany.

And she's holding a gift bag.

Ding-dong merrily on high.

CHAPTER 22

Tiffany Drops Off a Gift

I'm totally confused.

Tiffany is standing on my front porch, wearing a long, black fur coat that's glistening with tiny droplets of water where snowflakes must have landed and melted.

"What are you doing here?" I finally manage to ask.

"Well, that's not very...," Tiffany starts to say in her snotty voice, but then stops herself. She glances behind her at the fancy white SUV in my driveway. She sighs, turns back to me, and switches the gift bag under her other arm. "I'm on my way to church with my parents, but I need to give something to Papa Shortdough. May I please see him?"

"No!" I yell before I can catch myself. There's no way Tiffany can see him while he still thinks he's a superhero, or a finder of umbrellas or whatever.

"Why not?"

Too late I realize my mistake. I shut the door a crack more. I can still see Tiffany, but hopefully she can't see inside. "Because he's not here."

She frowns. "But he wasn't at his market, and I was told he was here."

"Who told you that?"

"Nick."

I almost growl. Talk about traitors!

"Come on, Poppie, this is heavy," she complains. She props the gift bag against the door frame, accidentally hitting the doorbell again.

DING DONG

She gives me that exasperated Tiffany face. "So, is Papa Shortdough here, or not?"

"Who wants to know?" Papa's voice booms from behind me.

I panic. He's walking towards us. Tiffany can't see him! How would I ever explain it?

Oh, so, yeah. My parents hypnotized him so he doesn't know who he is anymore. Yes, go ahead. Call the police. Arrest us all.

My parents are just trying to help me. I don't want to get them into trouble!

So, I do the only thing I can do in a situation like this. I slam the door in Tiffany's face.

Papa joins me in the front hall. He has an odd look on his face, but his eyes are twinkling and his eyelids blinking.

"Papa?" I stammer.

"Yes, Poppie?"

My eyes widen. "Is it really you?"

He chuckles. "Yes. Who else would I be?"

Mom, Dad, Berg, and Kale are standing in the front room. Papa has his back to them, so he can't see that they're all waving at me and shaking their heads.

Mom gives me a look. "Papa Shortdough just stopped by to say hi," she says too loudly.

I grimace. I'm guessing they haven't worked on lying yet in PI school.

"So, we invited him to stay for dinner," Dad adds.

My face brightens. I grab Papa's arm. "Oh, will you stay? Please? Pretty please?"

Kale walks up, slings his arm around my shoulders, and

laughs. "Come on, Papa, you know she won't stop until you say yes."

Papa grins. "Very true." He smiles at my parents. "Thank you for the invitation. I'd love to stay."

The doorbell rings again.

DING DONG

Oops. I totally forgot about Tiffany.

I pull open the door, smiling. "What do you know, Tiffany..."

I stop mid-sentence. Instead of Tiffany, I'm face to face with Miss Sweettarte. She's smiling brightly at me with fresh curls in her gray bob, red lipstick brightening her lips, and her arm laced tightly through her grandson's.

Nick chuckles. "Now you want to call me Tiffany? If I have a choice, I think I like Red better."

I shake my head. "No, no. Tiffany was just here and..." I peek around them, wondering if she's hiding in the bushes or if they pushed her off the porch. Not that I would blame them or anything.

Nick pretends to look under his feet. "Tiffany was here?"

Miss Sweettarte whacks Nick's arm. "Don't tease the poor darlin', Nick. It's Christmas Eve."

Nick ducks his head a bit, but grins. "Okay, Nams."

Ms. Sweettarte smiles at me. It's as warm as sunshine on a summer day. "Thank you, sweet Poppie darlin', for inviting us over for Christmas Eve dinner."

I quickly remember my manners. "I'm so happy you could come, Miss Sweettarte." I step back to let them in. "Please come in."

Miss Sweettarte steps into the front hall, and Papa Short-dough rushes forward.

"Sweetie! You're here!" he gushes, giving Miss Sweettarte a peck on the cheek. His smile is so huge that I've never seen so many happy crinkles near his eyes. He helps her out of her fluffy white coat.

"Papa, I'll take that," I offer.

He hands me her coat but doesn't even look at me. He's too busy beaming at Miss Sweettarte.

"You look as pretty as a sunrise on Christmas morning," he says.

And I have to agree. She's wearing a dusty pink velvet dress that gives her cheeks a rosy blush. Or maybe that's just from Papa's compliment.

Papa links his arm through Miss Sweettarte's and leads her into the living room, leaving Nick and I alone in the entry.

Thanks," I murmur, so only he can hear me. "You actually came through."

He opens his mouth to say something, but then closes it and shakes the snow off his head. He sighs. "It's probably my fault you think I'm this mean guy you can't trust." And for a split second he looks at me. I mean really looks at me. His eyes turn soft, like melted chocolate, and he leans towards me...

Am I about to get my first kiss?!

From Nick?!

But instead, he reaches out and tucks my braid over my shoulder. "I'm not really all that bad, Poppie, and I hope I can change your mind about me. Because I like you and think you're perfect just the way you are," he winks and adds, "*Kid*." He grabs my hand. "Come on. The rest of your plan is about to come true."

I let him lead me into the living room, but I don't know what to think. What is he saying? He likes me? Do I like him? He thinks I'm perfect just the way I am? Not twenty pounds lighter?

Just as I am?

Nick walks up to Papa. He releases my hand and hands Papa a gift bag. "This is for you. I think you're really going to like it so maybe you can open it now?"

"Okay," Papa says with a smile. "Thanks, Nick."

Papa reaches into the bag and pulls out a dark brown box with white cursive on the side.

His eyes grow wide.

I gasp.

It's beginning to look a lot like Christmas!

CHAPTER 23

Papa Is So Very Happy

"Where did you get this?" Papa asks, looks of confusion and elation battling for rights on his face. "I thought I lost it. I couldn't find it anywhere. Even Poppie and Kale helped me look."

Wait. This is Papa's box of chocolate?

And Nick had it all along?

He just told me that he wasn't *that* guy. Why would he steal Papa's chocolate? Papa gave him a job. Miss Sweettarte welcomed him into her home.

And I almost let him kiss me.

He's just as bad as I thought he was when I first met him.

I mumble some excuse about checking on dinner, and run into the kitchen.

The smell of sharp asiago and rich chicken fills the air, making my stomach growl, but I don't even feel hungry. If Nick is a bully and a thief, then what just happened in the front hall? Why did he seem sad when he thought I didn't trust him?

And why do I even care?!

Is it because I like him? Do I like Nick?

I sink onto a stool, and close my eyes. This is definitely not part of my plan.

"Need any help?"

I open my eyes to find Nick's chocolaty ones sparkling at me, so full of hope and… deceit?

I narrow my eyes. "Where did you get that box?"

He looks hurt. "You still don't trust me, do you?"

I don't answer right away. Do I trust him? He did get Miss Sweettarte here like he promised.

I sigh. "I want to. I really do."

He shrugs. "That's a good enough start." He plops onto the stool next to me. "As I was just telling Papa Shortdough, Tiffany was on the porch when Nams and I arrived. She said you slammed the door in her face." He chuckles. "Which sounds like you. Anyway, she said she had to go, but wanted to make sure Papa Shortdough got the box. I knew he'd be here if everything was going to plan so I took it from her."

So, Tiffany did steal the box! I was right!

Papa burst into the kitchen with Kale on his heels. He sets the box on the counter and looks at us, his face flushed.

"This is my box!" Papa shakes his head. "I wonder why Tiffany had it?"

Because she stole it.

"She said something about it being delivered to their restaurant by accident," Nick explains.

Papa nods his head. "That makes sense. I share delivery service with C'est La Ski. I must have accidentally left it near the stack of boxes I wanted to mail, and the delivery service took it."

Yeah. Right. And I no longer love junk food.

Miss Sweettarte's sugary Southern voice filters in from the living room. "Nick, darlin', will you please come here when you get a minute?"

"Sure thing, Nams," Nick calls back. He grins at us. "You should have seen her face when I told her we were invited to dinner. It was like Christmas came early." He stands and smooths out his pants, not making eye contact. "It's really nice to be around a big, happy family for the holiday since my parents were called up," he pauses and looks right at me. "So, thanks. It means a lot."

I watch him saunter out of the kitchen. Who knew Nick had a heart. A sweet heart it seems.

I frown. "What does he mean his parents were called up?"

"They're both in the military," Papa explains. "They just left on a year-long assignment."

Yikes. Right before Christmas.

"Will they get to come home and visit?" Kale asks.

Papa shakes his head and frowns. "Unfortunately, no. And they're a close family like you." He looks toward the living room. "I don't know if I should say this, but it's been hard on him."

Wow. I didn't even know.

Papa sniffs the air. "Something sure smells great in here."

Oh no! The chicken! I grab the potholders and open the oven, hoping there's not another disaster awaiting me. I exhale a sigh. The chicken is perfectly browned. No smoke. Nothing black. Nothing burned.

Whew.

Papa peeks over my shoulder. "Poppie, that looks delicious!"

"Clea made it," I admit.

He looks confused. "Is she here, too?"

I shake my head. "Not anymore."

I grab the rolls off the counter and put them in the oven. Papa suddenly notices the food surrounding him.

Santa's Cozy Chicken
Snowman Carrots
Reindeer Salad
Star Rolls
Chocolate Chimney Cake

His mouth gapes open. "Clea made all this?"

I smile proudly. "Yep. Along with the rest of your *Yum Yum* class."

Kale nudges me. "But only because of Poppie's plan."

Papa peels back the foil covering the *Chocolate Chimney*

Cake and peeks in.

"Those were cupcakes." I grimace. "Until I burned them."

Kale wraps his arm around my shoulder. "But you'd be so proud of her, Papa. She didn't give up because her recipe didn't go as planned." He grins. "She took your advice and just tweaked it!"

Papa grabs a cake piece, pops it in his mouth, and chews. He beams at me. "Delicious! And way better than the original, I bet."

"Kale made the salad and carrots," I brag. "And Li and Nacho made the rolls. We made it all from scratch. Our meal is a little healthy, a little treat, a smidge of tweaking, and a whole lot of love. Just like you taught us." I shrug, oddly feeling a little embarrassed. "We all wanted you to have a good Christmas Eve dinner."

Papa looks a little misty-eyed. "All my *Yum Yum* students worked together to create this beautiful meal?" He wipes his eyes with a beefy thumb and takes a deep breath. "And now Miss Sweettarte is here. It's all coming together, isn't it?" He raises a bushy eyebrow at me. "I wonder how that happened?"

I blush. "I hope you're not mad. I know you wanted to have dinner with Miss Sweettarte, and I wanted to make you happy again."

He tugs my braid. "Poppie, I am happy. And I don't think I could ever be mad at you." He scratches his chin. "But someday you'll have to tell me exactly how I got here because I sure don't remember." He chuckles. "Which means it must be a pretty good story." He gathers Kale and me in a hug. His muscular arms squash us tight. "Thank you. Thank you." His voice breaks, and I wonder if our sweet, bodybuilding baker is crying.

He squeezes us once more before letting go. He wipes his eyes, and gazes down at the box. "I still can't believe Tiffany found it."

I snort. "Found it? I still wonder if she took it."

"Now Poppie," Papa scolds. "We don't know that. The delivery truck probably took it from my restaurant with the boxes I had set to go out that day and then delivered it to them by accident like she said." He shrugs. "We'll probably never know, but the important thing is that I have the box again." He takes a deep breath. "And I guess there's only one way to find out if it's still in there."

He slowly opens the box, reaches inside, and pulls out a bar of chocolate.

I hold my breath.

He reaches in and pulls out another bar. He starts to reach in again, and then suddenly stops, a goofy smile on his face. I momentarily panic and wonder if he slipped into hypnosis again, but then he winks at me. He lifts out a small, blue velvet box, his goofy smile growing as huge as a sunflower unfolding in the sunlight.

"Is that it?" I squeal.

He nods. And without another word, he strides back into the front room with Kale and I on his heels.

Here comes Santa Claus, right to Miss Sweettarte's heart.

CHAPTER 24

The Best Christmas Eve EVER

P apa walks up to Miss Sweettarte and clears his throat. "Excuse me. May I have everyone's attention, please?"

Everyone stops talking and looks at him.

He smiles. "Thank you." I see a small bead of sweat roll down the side of his face. "First, I want to thank the wonderful Wellington family for inviting us all over for Christmas Eve dinner. Especially, Poppie, who I'm pretty sure had this all perfectly planned out." He turns to me and winks.

I blush.

"Second, I want to thank all of you for being my friends, and for supporting my market. You are the only ones who know that someone is trying to run me out, and I love that every single one of you has offered to help." He turns to my parents. "And I really appreciate what the two of you are doing to help me find out just who is causing all this trouble."

Kale punches me in the shoulder and whispers, "PI school."

Ohhh. The secret. The one my parents couldn't tell me. It was about Papa. They're learning to be private investigators to help him with his store! I grin. Like daughter like parents.

Papa inhales a deep breath, faces Miss Sweettarte, and takes her hand. "And, finally, I want to thank my sweetie for being here by my side this past year."

I hold my breath. Is he?

Papa smiles at Miss Sweetarte. "I have loved you since the day you galloped your little pony into town. I want to cook beautiful dinners for you, and spoil you with *Triple-Chocolate Cookies*, and spend the rest of our life talking by the firelight." He reaches into his pocket, pulls out the little blue box, and drops onto one knee.

OH MY GOSH! HE IS!

Papa's voice chokes a little when he asks. "Will you marry me, my southern belle?"

Miss Sweettarte breaks into a grin that's brighter than the star on top of our Christmas tree. "Goodness gracious, yes, you cutie-patooty! Of course, I'll marry you!"

Papa whoops, leaps up, and twirls her around in a hug.

Kale flings his arm over my shoulders. "Looks like your plan worked," he says with a grin.

I can't help but smile. He's right. It worked. My plan actually worked.

I knock my hip into his. "It took a few tweaks here and there, and a lot of help from you and our friends, but you're right. It did work."

Kale beams at me. "Never had a doubt." He gives my shoulder a squeeze, and then walks over to congratulate Papa and Miss Sweettaarte.

Mom sidles up to me. She tilts her head. "You okay?"

I nod. "More than okay. I can't believe this all worked out."

Mom laughs. "Of course, it worked! You're an amazing girl with wonderful gifts like kindness, spirit, and loads of determination. When you make a plan people can't help but follow you."

I smile, and give her a hug. "Thanks, Mom. Nothing would have worked if you and Dad hadn't gotten Papa here." I hug her again, and then have a thought. "How did you un-hypnotize him?"

She flutters her hands. "I was so lucky! When you went to answer the doorbell, I remembered that a man in a suit was ringing Papa's doorbell while we were hypnotizing him. I just had to un-hypnotize him when the doorbell was ringing, and it worked."

"Wait. Did you say a man in a suit?" This is a mountain town. I've only seen one person who wears a suit.

Mom nods. "Yes. We didn't answer the door, so I don't know who it was, but hopefully it was nothing important since we had to hustle Papa out of there."

I narrow my eyes. "I think he was the guy trying to convince Papa to sell his restaurant."

Mom frowns. "Are you sure?"

I shrug. "I don't know for certain, but I would definitely recognize him if I saw him again."

She nods. "Ok. Dad and I may need your help with this."

I raise my eyebrows. "Really? Even though I'm not a private investigator?"

She grins. "Of course! You have ways of getting people to go along with your plan. That is a great skill for an investigator to have."

I almost laugh out loud. If only she knew about Miss Icy talking her way into the C'est La Ski pantry.

"And I'm really impressed how you got everyone to work together for this dinner," she continues.

Oh no! The rolls!

"I'm going to check on dinner," I say, trying to sound all casual and not at all stressed. I don't want her to know something may be wrong. I told them I was going to cook and I don't want to mess this up.

"Do you need any help?" she asks.

"Not at all," I say a little too loudly. "You stay here and relax," I call over my shoulder as I race off to the kitchen, hoping I'm not too late.

But I am.

Smoke is curling around the oven in a grin. Again.

I grab potholders, pull open the oven, and pull out the rolls.

You've got to be kidding me! Li and Nacho's beautifully crafted rolls are all topped with a super lovely black crust.

Nick rushes into the kitchen behind me. "Is everything okay? You ran in here so fast I thought something may be wrong."

"Something is," I moan. I glare at the oven. "You are definitely out to get me," I growl. I gesture to the rolls. "Burned. Just like the pancakes. Just like the cookies. Just like the cupcakes."

Nick examines the rolls. "They're just a little burned."

I throw my hands in the air. "Who cares if it's a little or a lot! They're burned! They're ruined! They're inedible!"

Nick tilts his head. "It's okay. It's just rolls. We can just take the tops off. I bet the insides are still good."

I shake my head. "I can't do anything right."

Nick half-smiles, and says softly, "That's not true. You got us all together for Christmas Eve. That's very right. Who cares if we eat burnt rolls, or pancakes, or even food from a carton. The important thing is that we're all together." He grins. "Although I'm also pretty sure your oven is not a team player, and is *definitely* out to get you."

That makes me snort.

He chuckles.

And then I can't help it. I burst out laughing.

He's right. Here I am complaining about burnt rolls when that's not what's important. I wanted to learn to cook some healthy dishes, and I did. I wanted to make Christmas Eve dinner, and with the help of some amazing friends, I did. I wanted to help Papa so he could propose to Miss Sweettarte and they could live happily ever after, and I did. I haven't lost twenty pounds or had my first kiss, but that's okay. There's time for that.

I wipe my eyes. "Thanks, Nick. I needed that." I smile. "You're right. I just wanted to see Papa and Miss Sweettarte happy. And it is pretty cool that we're all here together on

Christmas Eve."

"Even me?" he asks. He raises an eyebrow. "Are you happy your old pal, Red, is here?"

I am happy he's here. I really am.

I pause. Should I tell him how I feel? Liking him is not part of my plan, but maybe it should be a last minute addition. A tweak to my plan.

Besides, what do I have to lose?

I look into Nick's warm chocolaty eyes. "Yes. I'm actually really glad you're here." My heart races. My hands feel clammy. But I continue. "Because... I think... I think I like you."

Nick looks startled for a split second, and then grins really, really big. His eyes grow soft. He tucks my braid behind my shoulder. He leans in...

My first kiss. IT'S ABOUT TO HAPPEN!

Nick leans in further, closes his eyes... and stops inches from my mouth.

Why?!

He presses his forehead to mine, and sighs. "I want to kiss you, Poppie. I really do." He exhales. "But I shouldn't."

My heart sinks. "Because I'm fat?" I whisper.

His eyes widen and he pulls his head back. "No! Why would you even say that?" He sighs. "You're perfect. You have a big..."

"Thighs?"

He shakes his head. "Poppie, stop. I was going to say a big heart, and a big personality, and a big, beautiful smile, and..." He gazes at me with those chocolaty eyes until a grin tugs at his lips. "Oh, what the heck," he says, leans in...

AND KISSES ME!

HE KISSES ME!

Nick Sweettarte kisses me! His soft lips taste like peppermint as they lightly press against mine, leaving me feeling tingly and warm.

He leans back and looks at me, a trace of fear in his eyes. "Was that okay?"

I giggle and blush, like a tiny schoolgirl. Me, huge towering Poppie Pie, giggling after her first kiss.

I nod. "Yes, that was more than okay." I giggle again, but then raise an eyebrow. "Wait, I thought you said you didn't want to kiss me?"

He looks shocked. "I never said I didn't want to. I just thought I shouldn't."

I tilt my head. "Why?"

Now it's his turn to blush. "When I told Nams I liked you, she insisted I take you out on a proper date before I even thought about kissing you." He grabs my hands. "So, what do you say? Will you go out on a proper date with me?" He grins wickedly, eyes sparkling. "I could even take you to C'est La Ski?"

"I'd love to go on a date with you anywhere but there," I laugh.

"Then how about Papa's Market?" he suggests.

I grin and smile. "I would like that."

Our first date will be where we first met. Plus, I have a feeling The Suit will be back, and Papa's going to need all his friends by his side.

Wait a minute. My eyes widen. "You told Nams you liked me?"

He grins. "From the moment I watched you run around and around like a lunatic in that revolving door, I liked you. Because you, Poppie Pie, are so sweet," he laughs and adds, "yet so salty. You are a perfect, irresistible mix."

My heart beats a little faster. "Really?"

He nods. Leans in, and kisses me again.

Well, what do you know? Boys do kiss fat girls.

Because we are irresistible. And perfect.

I like the sound of that.

FA LA LA LA LA la la la la.

Until next time... have fun cooking!

POPPIE'S TIPS FOR HEALTHY EATING

1. EAT ALL FOODS
Try to include Vegetable, Fruit, Whole Grain, and Protein at each meal! Healthy foods are full of vitamins, minerals, fiber, and energy you need daily!

2. EAT EVERY COLOR
Eat a variety of colors every day! The more colors you eat, the more good-for-you nutrients you give your body!

3. LOVE YOUR VEGGIES AND FRUITS
Fill at least half your plate with Fruits and Vegetables! They help you stay strong, fast, clever, healthy, and ready to have fun!

4. START SMALL
Take a smaller portion, or use a smaller plate! If you're not full, you can always go back for seconds!

5. EAT MINDFULLY
Instead of watching TV or your phone, really be there with your delicious food!
Try Papa's way: chew slowly, and savor every yummy bite!

RECIPES

◆ ◆ ◆

APPETIZERS

Smile Hour Appie

BREAKFASTS

Cheesy Salsa Burritos

Cinnamon Oats & Apples

Fluffy Pancakes with Fresh Berries

LUNCHES

Cornie Quinoa

Mozzie Tom Sammies

Papa's Favorite Vegetable Soup

Tuna, Berries & Greens

DINNER

Reindeer Salad

Santa's Cozy Chicken

Snowman Carrots

Star Rolls

DESSERTS

Papa's Triple-Chocolate Cookies

Chocolate Chip Love Cookies

Chocolate Chimney Cupcakes

PAPA'S TRIPLE-CHOCOLATE COOKIES

Papa finally gave me his recipe for these fudgy chocolate cookies with luscious white-chocolate and dark-chocolate chips. He said it can be our little secret.

Makes approximately 24 cookies

INGREDIENTS:

¾ cup (1 ½ sticks) unsalted Butter, softened

1 ¼ cups Sugar

2 Eggs

2 tsp Vanilla Extract

2 cups Flour

1/3 cup Unsweetened Cocoa Powder

1 tsp Baking Powder

¼ tsp Salt

1 cup Dark Chocolate Chips (Use 60% or Semi-Sweet Chocolate Chips)

¾ cup White-Chocolate Chips

INSTRUCTIONS:

1. Preheat oven to 350 degrees. Convect Bake works best for cookies!
2. Dump Butter into a large mixer bowl, and mix until light. Add Sugar and beat a few minutes until fluffy. May need to scrape down sides of bowl.
3. Add Eggs and Vanilla Extract, and mix, scraping down sides as needed.
4. Spoon Flour into measuring cup. Add Baking Powder and Salt. With mixer set on low, slowly add to bowl. Mix well.
5. Add Cocoa Powder, and mix well.
6. Stir in Dark and White Chocolate chips.
7. Drop balls (approximately the size of 2 Tbsp) about 2-inches apart on a nonstick cookie sheet. Bake 8-10 minutes, or until cookies begin to crack but are not completely set.
8. Let cool 5 minutes. Remove from tray.
9. Savor one, and feel your worries melt away!

SMILE HOUR APPIE

Guaranteed to make everyone smile! When you make this for your parents or friends, pretend you're in Spain with Nacho and call them tapas. Everyone will be so impressed you may never have to do dishes again!

Serves 4-6

INGREDIENTS:

20- 30 Crackers

6-8 ounces Cheese, cut into cracker-sized bites -*Try 2-3 types. I like cheddar, manchego, and gouda!*

2 cups Vegetables, sliced - *Try carrots, celery, edamame, red and green peppers, broccoli, or jicama!*

Fiesta Dip:

¼ cup Nonfat Greek Yogurt, plain

3 Tbsp Salsa

⅛ tsp Garlic Powder

INSTRUCTIONS:
1. Pull out a small bowl for the dip, and a large platter for the cheese and vegetables.
2. Slice Cheese and Vegetables.
3. Arrange Vegetables on one side of the platter, and Cheese and Crackers on the other. I like to make smiley faces, a heart, or even a Christmas tree!
4. Mix Yogurt, Salsa, and Garlic Powder until blended. Pour into the small bowl. If there's room on the platter, set the bowl next to the vegetables.
5. Serve, smile, and be APPIE! ☺

FLUFFY PANCAKES WITH FRESH BERRIES

I know you won't burn them. Light and fluffy all the way!

Makes 12 pancakes

INGREDIENTS:

1 cup All-Purpose Flour

½ cup White Whole-Wheat Flour

1 Tbsp Sugar

2 tsp Baking Powder

¾ tsp Salt

1 cup Nonfat Milk

2 Tbsp Greek Yogurt, plain, nonfat

1 Tbsp Olive Oil

1 Egg

1 tsp Vanilla Extract

1 cup Raspberries, Blueberries or Strawberries (or all 3)

¼ cup Walnuts, chopped (optional)

INSTRUCTIONS:

1. Wash Berries. If nothing is in season, buy frozen blueberries. Thaw by pouring berries into a small pot, and warm over medium-low heat.

2. Add dry ingredients (Flour, White Whole-Wheat Flour, Sugar, Baking Powder, Salt) to a large mixing bowl. Whisk to mix.

3. Make hole in the center of dry ingredients, add wet ingredients (Milk, Yogurt, Oil, Egg, Vanilla), and whisk together. Do not overmix, or your pancakes may not be fluffy. The Batter may be lumpy.

4. Heat griddle or skillet over medium-low heat. Drop by spoonful. Cook until you see tiny bubbles on the surface, then flip over and finish cooking the other side.

5. Serve stacked high with lots of berries.

CHEESY SALSA BURRITOS

Quick and easy breakfast! Or make ahead,
store in the fridge, and heat to go!

Makes 4 burritos

INGREDIENTS:

Homemade Salsa:
½ cup Tomatoes, diced
2 Tbsp Sweet or Red Onion, diced
Salt, to taste
Dried Cilantro, to taste (optional)
Add 2 Tbsp Strawberries if in season (optional)

4 Eggs
1 Tbsp Milk, nonfat
Onion Powder, dash
Black Pepper, pinch
1 tsp Olive Oil
4 Tortillas - Whole-wheat/Corn blend, or Flour, soft taco size
½ cup Cheddar Cheese, shredded

INSTRUCTIONS:
1. Make salsa by mixing Tomatoes and Onions (and Strawberries if in season) in a small bowl. Add a dash of Salt or Cilantro if desired, to taste. Set aside and allow the flavors to meld while you prepare the rest.
2. Crack Eggs into a bowl. Add Milk, Onion Powder, and Pepper. Whisk thoroughly.
3. Heat nonstick skillet over medium heat. Add Olive Oil to coat bottom of pan. Add egg mixture and cook. Stir constantly until they are no longer runny and cooked through.
4. Wrap tortillas in a towel. Microwave for 10-20 seconds to warm.
5. Scoop ¼ of the eggs into the center of each tortilla. Sprinkle with ¼ of cheese and salsa. Enjoy!

CINNAMON OATS & APPLES

Perfectly delicious and filling on a chilly day!

Serves 2

INGREDIENTS:

1 cup nonfat Milk

¾ cup Water

1 cup old-fashioned Oats

1 tsp Cinnamon

1 Apple, chopped

2 Tbsp Walnuts, chopped

INSTRUCTIONS:

1. Boil Milk and Water over medium heat. Watch carefully so it doesn't boil over! When it starts to bubble and boil on the sides, stir in Oats and Cinnamon. Decrease heat to low simmer, and cook for approximately 5-10 minutes, stirring occasionally

2. Spoon cooked oats into a bowl. Top with apples and Walnuts, and enjoy!

CHOCOLATE CHIP LOVE COOKIES

Add in your secret ingredient to make this your own amazing recipe! I added a * to the additions you can tweak. Remember to write a good thought about the person on a napkin before you serve them your cookie!

Makes 24 cookies

INGREDIENTS:

¾ cup Pecans, lightly toasted

¾ cup Brown Sugar, packed

½ cup granulated Sugar

12 Tbsp unsalted Butter, softened

2 Eggs

2 tsp Vanilla Extract

2 ¼ cup Flour

1 teaspoon Baking Soda

½ teaspoon Salt

12 oz (2 cups) Chocolate Chips (I like half 50-60% dark and half semi-sweet)

½ cup Your Secret Ingredient (Cherries? Coconut? Candies?)

INSTRUCTIONS:
1. Preheat oven to 350 degrees. Convect Bake works best for cookies!
2. Lightly toast nuts. Let cool while assembling other ingredients.
3. In a large mixing bowl, whip Brown Sugar, Sugar, and Butter on Medium-High speed until light and fluffy. Approximately 2-4 minutes.
4. Add Eggs and Vanilla. Mix well, scraping down sides of bowl as needed.
5. Measure out Flour. Add Baking Soda and Salt. Dump in bowl. Add Chocolate Chips. Blend until dough forms.
6. Mix in nuts. The mixer will crush them into smaller pieces.
7. Stir in Your Secret Ingredient. ☺
8. Drop balls (approximately the size of 2 Tbsp) about 2-inches apart on a nonstick cookie sheet. Bake 7-10 minutes. Don't overcook!
9. Let cool 5 minutes, write your good thought or compliment on a napkin, and serve up some happiness!

PAPA'S FAVORITE VEGETABLE SOUP

Hearty and cozy warm on a cold day. Just like Papa's Market!

Serves 6-8

INGREDIENTS:

1 Tbsp Olive Oil

1 Onion, medium, chopped

5 Garlic Cloves, chopped

7 cups Chicken (or Vegetable) Broth

1 Tbsp Dried Basil

1 tsp Italian Seasoning

1 tsp Thyme

½ tsp Pepper

¼ - ½ tsp Red Pepper Flakes

¾ pound Red Potatoes, cut into 1 inches pieces

2 cup Carrots, cut into bite sized pieces

1 - 15 oz. can Cannellini White Beans

1 - 14.5 oz can Fire Roasted Tomatoes, diced

1 - 15 oz can Lima Beans (or 10 oz. frozen)

INSTRUCTIONS:

1. Place large pot over Medium heat. Add Olive Oil, and heat. Add Onion and saute for 5 minutes. Add Garlic

and saute 2 minutes.

2. Add rest of ingredients: Broth through Lima Beans. Bring to a simmer. Cover partially with a lid, and let simmer for at least 2 hours.

MOZZIE TOM SAMMIES

Easy, yummy, and a groovy-cool name! What else do you need?

Serves 4

INGREDIENTS:

4 slices Whole-Wheat Bread, or rolls
1-2 Tbsp Balsamic Glaze
1-2 Tbsp Olive Oil
4-6 ounces Part-Skim Mozzarella, sliced
2 large Tomatoes, cut into 8 slices
4-8 large, fresh Basil Leaves

INSTRUCTIONS:
1. Toast Bread.
2. In a small dish, mix Olive Oil and Balsamic Vinegar. Drizzle on one side of toast, or use as a dipping sauce.
3. Top each piece of drizzled toast with Mozzarella, then Basil, and then Tomato.
4. Cut each sandwich in half, and serve.

TUNA, BERRIES, & GREENS

So easy! So colorful! So wonderful! I want to eat it now.

Serves 4

INGREDIENTS:

4 cups fresh Greens, chopped into strips -*Try a mixture with Spinach, Kale, and Green Leaf!*

2 pouches (3 ounces each) Albacore Tuna - *Some varieties are flavored, like ranch or spicy. Try them!*

½ cup Walnuts, coarsely chopped

1 cup Blueberries

1 Apple, sliced

Olive Oil **or** your favorite Dressing

INSTRUCTIONS:
1. Mix Greens, Walnuts, Berries. Divide among four plates. Top with tuna.
2. Drizzle with Olive Oil, or your favorite light dressing.
3. Serve with freshly cut apple slices on the side.

CORNIE QUINOA

A funny name! A fun lunch! I love taking it to school.

Serves 4

INGREDIENTS:
- ¾ cup Quinoa
- 2 cups Chicken or Vegetable Broth
- 2 tablespoons Olive Oil
- 1 teaspoon Cumin
- ½ teaspoon Chili Powder
- ½ teaspoon Garlic Powder
- ½ teaspoon Salt
- 1 ½ teaspoon Lime Juice
- 1 small Red Bell Pepper, chopped
- 1 cup Baby Tomatoes, sliced in half
- 1 (15oz) can Corn, drained
- 1 (15 oz) can Black Beans, drained and rinsed

INSTRUCTIONS:

1. Place Quinoa and Broth in a medium saucepan. Bring to a boil and simmer, covered, for 15-20 minutes, or until liquid is mostly absorbed and each quinoa grain is translucent. Let sit 5 minutes.
2. While quinoa cooks, whisk Olive Oil, Cumin, Chili Powder, Garlic Powder, Salt and Lime together to make a dressing.
3. Mix Red Bell Pepper, Tomatoes, Corn, and Black Beans into cooked quinoa. Add dressing. Toss until mixed.
4. Best if refrigerated for 30 minutes or longer, but also tasty if still warm.
5. Really yummy and so good for you served over a bed of spinach, or wrapped in a tortilla for your lunch!

CHOCOLATE CHIMNEY CUPCAKES

A mistake turned fabulous!

Makes 12 cupcakes

INGREDIENTS:

2 Tbsp Olive Oil

3 Tbsp Greek Yogurt, nonfat plain

½ cup Brown Sugar, packed

2 Eggs

1 tsp Vanilla Extract

5 Tbsp unsweetened Cocoa Powder

1 cup + 3 Tbsp White Whole Wheat Flour

¼ cup Flour

1 teaspoon Baking Soda

¼ teaspoon Salt

1 cup Buttermilk (OR 1 Tbsp Vinegar + 1 cup Milk)

¾ cup Dark Chocolate Chips (50-70%)

Optional: Raspberries, Bananas, Vanilla Ice Cream

INSTRUCTIONS:
1. Preheat oven to 350 degrees.
2. Place cupcake liners in muffin pan, or spray with cooking spray.
3. Make buttermilk if you don't have it by adding 1

Tbsp Vinegar to 1 cup Nonfat Milk and let it sit a few minutes to curdle.

4. Mix Oil and Yogurt in a large mixing bowl on low speed. Add Brown Sugar, and mix until blended.

5. Add Egg and Vanilla. Mix thoroughly, scraping down sides of bowl as needed.

6. Mix Cocoa, Flours, Baking Soda, and Salt. Add ¼ to bowl and mix. Add ½ of Buttermilk to bowl and mix. Add rest of cocoa mixture and mix. Add rest of buttermilk, and mix until everything is incorporated.

7. Add Dark Chocolate Chips, and gently mix in on low.

8. Divide batter among cupcakes, filling the cups 2/3 full.

9. Bake for 10-15 minutes, or until middles are no longer jiggly.

10. Cool cupcakes.

11. Serve however you like! Whole cupcakes, or cut into pieces, and served with ice cream, raspberries, and bananas!

SANTA'S COZY CHICKEN

Rich and delicious, just like Santa makes for Mrs. Claus!

Serves 4

INGREDIENTS:

4 Chicken Breasts

4 oz. Greek Yogurt, nonfat

½ cup Asiago, grated

½ tsp Salt

1 tsp Garlic Powder

½ tsp Black Pepper

INSTRUCTIONS:

1. Preheat oven to 375 degrees.
2. Line baking dish with aluminum foil, and spray with cooking spray. Place Chicken in dish.
3. Combine Yogurt, Cheese, and Spices. Spread over top of chicken.
4. Bake 35-45 minutes, or until the chicken has cooked through, and topping is browned.

SNOWMAN CARROTS

*Don't leave them out on Christmas Eve or the reindeer
will nibble them all up!*

Serves 4

INGREDIENTS:

2 cups Carrots, peeled and cut into 1-inch slices

½ Tbsp Olive Oil

2 Tbsp Water

⅛ tsp Salt

1 tsp Raspberry Vinegar

1 tsp Honey

INSTRUCTIONS:
1. In large saucepan, combine Carrots, Olive Oil, Water, and Salt. Simmer, partially covered, until tender, about 15 minutes.
2. Turn off heat. Add Vinegar and Honey. Toss to coat carrots, and serve.

REINDEER SALAD

This is Rudolph's favorite meal. I think you'll love it, too!

Serves 4

INGREDIENTS:

2 cups Spinach, cut into strips, loosely packed
2 Tbsp Asiago Cheese, shredded
½ Apple, diced
¼ cup Pomegranate Seeds, or Blueberries
¼ cup Walnuts, chopped

Vinaigrette:
1 Tbsp Champagne Vinegar
½ Tbsp Raspberry Balsamic Vinegar
½ Tbsp Honey
1-2 Tbsp Olive Oil, to taste
Salt, to taste

INSTRUCTIONS:
1. Toss Spinach, Asiago, Apple, Pom Seeds, and Walnuts together.
2. Whisk ingredients to make Vinaigrette.
3. Right before serving, add **1- 2 Tbsp** vinaigrette to salad and toss. Refrigerate the rest of dressing to use another time.

STAR ROLLS

There's nothing dreamier than the smell of fresh rolls baking. And you made them! Be sure to start them 2 hours before you want to eat.

Makes 12 rolls

INGREDIENTS:

1 cup Water

½ cup Oatmeal, quick or old-fashioned

¾ Tbsp Butter

1 ¼ tsp Dry Yeast

¼ cup Warm Water (110 degrees)

¼ cup Molasses

1 tsp Salt

2 ⅓- ½ cups Flour

INSTRUCTIONS:
1. Bring 1 cup of Water to a boil in a medium saucepan. Stir in Oats and Butter. **Let sit for 1 hour.**
2. Soak Dry Yeast in ¼ cup Warm Water (110 degrees) for 5 minutes. Watch the yeast dissolve and the bubbles rise!
3. Stir yeast mixture until dissolved. Add to a stand mixer bowl, then add Molasses, Salt, and Oat mixture, and mix with dough hook. Add 2 ⅓ cups flour. Dough should stick to the bowl a bit, but not stick to your fingers. Do not make the dough too dry. You can add up to another ¼ cup flour if excessively sticky. Knead with dough hook on medium for 8 minutes.
4. Roll into 12 ball-shapes. Place into muffin tin sprayed with cooking spray. **Let rise in a warm place for 30-60 minutes.**
5. Preheat oven to 375 degrees. Bake 10-12 minutes.

ABOUT THE AUTHOR

Suzanne Brown is a registered dietitian, wellness coach, food blogger, and author who loves every food from cookies to spinach!

She's a certified lover of life who lives at 8,000 feet in the Colorado mountains with her husband, two teenage kids, two dogs, and two horses. If they're not hiking, running, snowshoeing, or getting lost on a Jeep trail, they're exploring other playgrounds around the world - like skydiving over a volcano in Chile, swimming with elephants in Thailand, and mountain biking in Zimbabwe.

Suzanne holds dual degrees in Human Biology and Clinical Nutrition, and for the past 25 years has used her enthusiasm to teach teens and adults how to nurture a healthy and happy relationship with food. She loves teaching clients about moderation, mindful eating, and how to bake a super-rich chocolate cake at altitude.

She's also the author of **The Night Before Christmas in Ski Country** and **I'm With Anxious**.

Check out the next *Poppie Pie and The Yum Yum Club* book will release, as well as more recipes, tips and fun at:

SBtheRD.com

INSTAGRAM @SBtheRD   FACEBOOK @SBRD